I Want to Be Here

Conquering anxiety at its source to live with presence and peace at work and home

Joe Coleman

Coleman Insights Ink

Library of Congress Control Number: 2025902462

ISBN (Hardcover): 979-8-9919185-0-3
ISBN (Paperback): 979-8-9919185-1-0
ISBN (eBook): 979-8-9919185-3-4

Published by Coleman Insights Ink
San Clemente, California

Book Cover by Yucy Fang

Contents

Introduction

I don't want to be here. This meeting. My office. The dinner table. The neighborhood barbecue. What happens if the many "heres" in your life are the places you don't want to be? What if your "here" causes stress, anxiety, or even despair?

Maybe you wake up some mornings, or even every morning, with a weight on your shoulders and you just want to be free. Maybe your potential at work is stifled by your apprehension of falling short of expectations or fear of taking risks and ending up embarrassed. Maybe you've had one too many days where your anxieties have colored your interactions with the people you care about the most, weighing not just you down but your loved ones as well.

A common thread connects all these situations and more. There is a source that fuels their persistence. You have a story that's led you to this moment. You've struggled, perhaps a little and perhaps much more. But you want tomorrow to be different and believe it can be. That's why you're reading. You're here to learn something valuable you can apply in facing down a challenge that we all struggle with in different forms.

Several years ago, I found myself at a crossroads where the anxiety could have turned debilitating, holding me back from the life I was meant to live. Instead of stepping into the void, I took a different path - a longer road. Though the overall trajectory has been upward, there have been peaks and valleys. I'll recount that journey here and the lessons I've learned. The path led to the realization of a core insight concerning the source of anxiety and to develop a system to stand strong against it. I wrote this book to share the strategy and system with you. The discovery draws from my experience as a senior leader in the technology industry, managing the significant demands of long hours, intense competition, and an often cutthroat environment. It was also formed from years of research and deep study on topics ranging from psychotherapy to neuroscience. And as I've shared my story with others, they have shared their stories in return, contributing to this book's collective wisdom.

The first two chapters recount my story and the critical insight I uncovered. They lay the foundation for the system built on top of it. The remaining chapters identify how we can all apply the core strategy at work and home for maximum success in our battle against stress and anxiety. Through these later chapters, we'll unpack stories from others that provide sources of inspiration, as well as cautionary tales that bring the process to life. While my story begins with a focus on work, I spend just as much time on applications at home, as ultimately the two are inextricably linked, with our anxieties often transferring between these two states.

With so many other books that address the challenges posed by stress and anxiety, why pick this one? In trying to solve my anxiety challenge, I've read dozens of books on the topic and hundreds of others on related subjects. The challenge I found is that most approaches focus on implementing coping mechanisms once the anxiety has already surfaced. Many of these coping strategies can help, but if you don't address the source of your anxiety, management of the symptoms won't lead to a lasting resolution. Once anxiety makes an appearance, you're fighting an uphill battle, already having ceded the higher ground. And even if the coping mechanisms are effective, you've only put a Band-Aid on what's a deeper wound. When you've completed this book, you'll understand the source of your stress and anxiety and know how to move forward.

While our focus is to attack anxiety at its source, I also have a bonus for you. There is one scenario we'll use as a frequent example, which relates to how anxiety manifests at work and sometimes outside of work as well. That situation is anxiousness when speaking. And I'm not just talking about public speaking in front of hundreds or thousands of people; I'm also talking about speaking in a small group meeting or even sitting down with a single coworker, friend, or someone you're meeting for the first time one-on-one. If you ever feel anxious in these situations and if those feelings cause you to lose your breath as you speak, for your voice to fail, for your heart to race, or for you to forget your words, I'll share a technique that, when paired with the more significant approach of addressing the source of anxiety, will free you from those challenges. That technique shows up between Chapters 8 and 9, but consider it just the bonus, as our primary purpose is to go after the heart of the problem. As this is a long trail I have walked before, I'll act as your guide, but the journey is one we are taking together.

Chapter One

The Secret Struggle

I was in tree-lined Palo Alto, a part of Northern California where the weather is always beautiful and the tech industry that permeates the city is discretely tucked into the idyllic surroundings. A Massachusetts native, I had traveled west to be part of the special time in history when many of the brightest minds from around the world converged on this picturesque place, Silicon Valley. I was in my late 20s, working at my dream job, having climbed from a humble start to a leadership position at one of the premier technology companies in the world. I had the career, a wonderful wife, and even made a few close friends in my new home.

Yet something was wrong today. If I'm honest, something had been wrong for longer than that. But today was different. Something was *really* wrong. As I sat there at my desk, in the middle of an otherwise ordinary workday, I could feel my chest tightening and a sharp pain spreading. The feeling had been there before, but it was more intense now and escalating rapidly. I began sweating as if I had just finished an intense workout. My heart raced. Darkness clouded my vision and swallowed me up.

As I felt myself losing the battle to sustain my consciousness, my head involuntarily dropped to the desk. This couldn't be happening. I was having a heart attack in the middle of a random workday while just sitting there!

My conscious state returned. I don't think I was out for long, but this was a nightmare. Not just because of the physical symptoms I was experiencing, it was also a nightmare of embarrassment. I was a physically fit person, one of the younger people on the team, known for being strong, sharp, and capable. Was this the moment I had been dreading when the true nature of my strength was exposed? Did this mark the end of what I had worked years to achieve? And what would I do just to get out of this moment? Was someone calling an ambulance? Was I going to have to be carried out of here on a stretcher? No, it was okay. The severity of the symptoms had subsided. I just needed a few minutes to collect myself. I still needed to get out of here, but *I* could get myself out of here.

Thank God I didn't need an ambulance, but had anyone seen what was going on? I looked around. Somehow, everyone was still working as usual. Maybe they saw my head go down, but if they did, they must have assumed that I was frustrated by something or just taking a moment. That happens. While my body had regained semi-normal function, I still felt severely weakened and the pain in my chest remained strong. I waited a few more minutes to ensure I had the strength to collect myself and leave. I would drive to the nearest hospital and go from there. I stood up. Step one was complete, and I was still okay. I walked over to my boss's office. Not venturing in too far, I quickly told her I felt awful and needed to finish the day from home. This declaration was not typical for me, given I've never taken a sick day, but my announcement didn't raise any suspicions other than general wishes to "feel better soon." She returned to what she was doing as I slipped away.

I felt capable enough to drive, so I cautiously ventured to the nearest Palo Alto hospital. I checked into the emergency room and told the staff I believed that I had just had a heart attack. For them, the admission wasn't cause for alarm, as I was consigned to the waiting area with an air of routine. Eventually, my turn arrived and I began a battery of tests, including a physical examination, a blood pressure test, a blood sample for analysis, an electrocardiogram or EKG, and others. After a couple of hours of bouncing between tests and waiting, the doctor came to explain the results. I was ready for the news. I knew what had happened. Yet, there was no graveness on his face. He looked me in the eyes and, instead of declaring the diagnosis I was expecting, he told me that I was fine. There was nothing wrong with me. I hadn't had a heart attack.

I was puzzled. I knew *something* happened and that it was definitely *not* good. As I waited for an explanation, the doctor offered that it was probably a panic attack. A panic attack!? That news was more shocking than the prognosis of a near-death experience. These physical manifestations couldn't have simply resulted from my over-active imagination. What about the intense chest pain? The sweating? The heart palpitations? I didn't stay isolated in my house for fear of going outside. *Those* are the people who have panic attacks, right? Yet, that was the only explanation he had for me. He went on to say that he was prescribing me Prozac, a medication to alter my mental state so

I could deal with the anxieties my work presented. He sent me on my way.

How did I get here? There is a story of how I arrived at this junction in my life, which I will first briefly share. The rest of the book details the principles that allowed me to move ahead. If applied, these principles enable us all to conquer the source of stress and anxiety.

***

I was always a strong student academically, but my future wasn't shaped with much thought. I knew I was going to college, but I didn't have a list of stretch schools and safety options or do any meaningful research on the range of choices. I didn't have a career in mind. I didn't even do any preparation for my SATs, which is surprising considering that I completed every homework assignment, studied for every quiz, and prepared for every test that would form the basis of my grades.

Why did I attend to the smaller things while leaving the more significant matters unplanned? It was part ignorance and part practicality. I come from a modest background. I tell my kids now the harrowing story of how, growing up, my family of five survived sharing a single small bathroom. They return my gaze with looks of astonishment. I knew that if I wanted to go to college, I had to pay for it, and I wasn't willing to take on massive debt to make that happen. But beyond being practical, I was also ignorant of the importance of college selection on your career. I mean, calculus is calculus, right? Economics is economics. The laws of these subjects don't change based on learning them in a 100-year-old building with ivy growing on the walls. I *may* have been a bit naïve.

Based on a brochure I picked up in my high school's gymnasium, I chose a state college about 40 minutes from my hometown. This twist of fate turned out to be one of those "non-choice choices" that I wouldn't trade for anything. I met my future wife and many of my closest lifelong friends at the school. However, as I pursued a business career, I realized that colleges *were* a differentiator when it came to job opportunities. The open doors that a top-tier institution enables would need to be pried open.

The realization wasn't discouraging. It led me to operate with a chip on my shoulder that served to drive me. I believed I could rise to the top, and if it took more work to make that happen, I would be up to the challenge. I began to develop what I refer to as an underdog mindset. I pictured a world with the odds stacked against me. That's the positive interpretation, and it's true that a "me vs. the world" mentality has driven my work ethic. Though if I'm honest with myself, my underdog mentality also likely had shades of an inferiority complex that people in business refer to as "imposter syndrome."[1]

After graduating, my first job was at a market research company in Massachusetts, serving clients in the technology industry. The company was small, with about 35 people. My bosses had PhDs and went to schools like MIT. In addition, it seemed like every one of our clients graduated from Harvard Business School, followed by a two-year stint at McKinsey (the famous management consulting company). It was a bit intimidating. But while there was an undercurrent of apprehension, my underdog side was alive, and I was ready to prove myself.

This period was during the 2007 and 2008 financial crisis, and our business took a big hit as clients reined in spending. I had my first experience of layoffs a few months into my employment. I remember our Chief Operating Officer going to the offices on either side of me, laying off those people but sparing me. The difficult climate had an interesting implication for me; it opened doors. I was an affordable new college graduate who demonstrated promise and was working hard. The business was declining and needed to over-deliver with fewer resources. It suddenly didn't matter what my pedigree was. What mattered was whether I could do the job. And I could.

I began to be relied on for advanced analysis, to shape client deliverables, and to manage client communications. I was promoted multiple times in my first two years. The business stabilized, and I felt like a key contributor to our success. Everything seemed to be going well on the outside. Yes, I had my moments of self-doubt, but who didn't? I was moving forward, being entrusted with more, and receiving great feedback. Yet, something was happening on the inside, and frighteningly, it was gaining steam.

Anxiety had begun seeping into me like a virus. Following the promotions, I began experiencing tightness in my chest and strange sensations of being on the verge of losing consciousness. I would have an underlying sense of impending doom through these episodes. I eventually visited a doctor to describe my experience. After an examination, she assured me I was in good physical health and confirmed my suspicion that my symptoms were likely stress-related. She had some suggestions, like disabling e-mail push notifications from my phone, which I did. The diagnosis was a relief. Just a little bit of everyday work stress. Nothing to be overly concerned about.

After three and a half years, I opted to join a much larger company operating in the same space. They aspired to build out their technology practice in the California Bay Area, so my fiancée and I moved from New England to California. While I was excited and believed I could do the job well, there was an underlying question: "Am I going to be exposed on this bigger stage?" Sure, I was successful in a small business with a couple dozen people, but this company operated globally with significantly greater resources. Despite my hesitations, the dynamics played out much like the first company. I advanced quickly and gained a reputation as one of the top performers and as an up-and-coming leader.

As we settled into our new life in Northern California, I was confident my past anxiety symptoms would subside. After all, I was growing in my career, moving up, and learning new things. I was getting stronger in my capabilities, so it only made sense that any stresses I felt would ease as I gained confidence. Yet, to my disappointment and growing concern, these symptoms seemed to be gaining momentum. It felt like I was on the verge of something "happening," as each occurrence brought me closer to some unseen breaking point.

The stress had multiple origins. The pressure of the client deliverables and deadlines loomed large. I recognized that one failed project jeopardized the potential for future business. There was the regular occurrence of layoffs and the continual threat of more to come. Also, presentations were a particularly acute source of stress. Public speaking is commonly cited as one of the top fears of the adult population. Surveys have found that people are more afraid of speaking in public than death.[2] Yet the reward for my good work was that I was expected to do just that.

I'm an introvert, and my default mode is to be silent and take things in. My predispositions were coupled with the pressure I would put on myself. I had the unhelpful tendency to label different presentations in my mind as "the biggest moment in my career." According to me, "biggest career moments" happened pretty frequently. In many ways, this assessment was accurate. The presentation is where the rubber meets the road. All the good work in the world doesn't matter if you can't communicate it effectively and, in my case, get people to see the value and act on the findings presented. And the moments *were* getting bigger. If I started out presenting to our team internally and did well, it would lead to a presentation with our clients. If that went well, they would bring us in front of their senior management. If phone discussions were promising, we'd travel to present in their executive boardrooms.

The problem was that, while I was having success, I was just trying to survive — to get through those moments. Leading up to them, I would start to instill a belief that my career was hanging in the balance. After they were completed, I didn't feel a sense of momentum and readiness to go again. I only felt relief. Each time I was asked to present something, the request itself would generate an immediate moment of panic in my mind. It got to a point where just *watching* someone else deliver a presentation gave me a low-level sense of anxiety, as I pictured myself in their place.

Despite the hurdles, I was moving forward. Still, it didn't *feel* like I had "made it" yet. It felt a bit like I was looking in from the outside. My clients, Google, Dropbox, HP, Intel, and others, had these incredible campuses I would visit. There were private chefs, workers zipped around office hallways on scooters, and dessert carts would roam common spaces. They had fitness facilities, soccer fields, laundry services, and the famed nap pods. We would get lunch in their cafeterias, and I marveled that you could choose from sushi to barbecue and everything in between. I learned about the stock options and bonuses these companies gave out. Even the water bottles with their logos printed on the outside impressed me. It was exciting to be in the middle of the tech industry, but it also felt like I was just a visitor. I was working *with* some of the biggest names in technology, but I wanted to work *for* those companies.

In 2015, my opportunity came to join a marquee technology company. VMware isn't a household name, as it sells software used in data centers rather than offering consumer products. Still, the company is revered for its track record of innovation and regularly ranks as one of the best places to work in the country. Their campus in Palo Alto is, in my mind, the most stunning headquarters in Silicon Valley, with modern buildings tucked into a forest setting with features like turtle ponds. I should clarify that I "sort of" had the chance to join this tech luminary, but I wasn't given the job immediately. VMware had been one of my main accounts. My client brought me on as a contractor, with the potential to join as a full-time employee down the line. They knew me and my work but still wanted me to prove it. No problem.

Well, there *was* one problem. The anxiety had continued to gain momentum. I had persisted in positioning more and more "biggest moments in my career," and here was another "biggest" right in front of me. Except this wasn't just one moment. I had a 12-month contract that represented *innumerable* moments, any of which could be the difference between my acceptance or rejection. If rejected, my label would read, "Couldn't cut it in the big leagues." Facing this challenge would take a lot, and I knew the stress was already getting to me. I recognized that something inside me needed restoration to make this undertaking sustainable. A break would surely do the trick.

I had three days between ending my most recent job and joining VMware. I decided to do something I never did before: take a short getaway alone. I had been married for a couple of years and did everything with my wife, but I figured that some solitude would reinstate the peace I was lacking. I drove a few hours north to visit Crater Lake, an almost surreal location in southern Oregon with a pristine, circular body of water that formed from the collapse of a volcano thousands of years ago, which slowly filled with crystal-clear water. I biked around the entirety of the lake. I went golfing at my hotel and barely saw another person on the course. I decided to try a massage for the first time (mainly because that seemed like the quintessential activity to combat stress). The trip was fun. It was peaceful. I thought it was the therapeutic experience I needed. Yet, while I had rested and reset, I had changed nothing in my approach.

I returned and jumped into my new role at VMware. Some companies don't create an easy way to distinguish between contractors and regular employees; this is not the case at VMware. The employee badges are white and include your name and personal photo. The contractor badges are similar, except they have a thick red stripe running across them, reminiscent of a scarlet letter. If it's not enough to distinguish you in the physical world as "not one of us," every e-mail is accompanied by a "c" moniker (for "contractor") to ensure your identification in every digital interaction.

I took on the challenge as any underdog would, by putting in the work. As a contractor, I was paid for 40 hours of work per week, yet I stayed at the office for 11 hours each day to match what my boss was doing, then put in time at home to ensure no one was outdoing me. When my boss noticed my schedule, she told me she only had the budget to cover the 40 hours I was under contract for and no more. I told her not to worry, as my weekly timecard would reflect 40 hours, regardless of how much time I was really putting in.

The hard work didn't take long to pay off. While my new company's talent level was elevated, my ability to distinguish myself was the same as it had been previously. Less than two months into a 12-month contract, they offered me the full-time role of Director, a highly unusual transition for someone operating in a contractor capacity. They gave me a team that included people previously giving me direction as their vendor. Some of those reporting to me were ten to twenty years older and had advanced degrees. Still in my 20s, I was one of the youngest directors in a company valued at over $30 billion, a valuation that would more than double in a few years. They gave me a generous salary, stock allocation, and perks like an office in a mostly open floor plan setting.

Now, I was working in Silicon Valley, where it's not uncommon for 20-somethings to run multi-billion-dollar companies. I was nowhere near that level of success, but I was working for a dream company, making more money than I would have thought possible at the peak of my career, and I was considered a leader at a company that had access to the best talent in the world. On the outside, I had made it. Yet, on the inside, the war was being waged.

I may have been in charge, but I didn't feel I was in control. I believed that some of my team looked at me with skepticism. I gave voice to their thoughts in my mind: "Who is this kid with zero pedigree now telling me what to do?" All the pressures I felt previously only deepened. Yes, it was the stress of deliverables, presentations, and management, but my anxiousness began appearing in new ways and seemingly relaxed settings. I started experiencing these anxiety symptoms of chest tightening, feelings of impending doom, and a sense that I was heading towards losing consciousness by simply sitting down in a meeting with a single other person.

People don't know what's going on inside you, so I was able to hold it together in most situations. My coworkers likely had no clue I was fighting this sensation back, but something was getting closer. Then, one day, it arrived. There was no particular event or circumstance that I can recall which triggered the panic attack. I believe it was simply the culmination of all the accumulated stress and anxiety that had been building for years and had accelerated in recent weeks. My body had had enough, and it shut down.

A panic attack is not an experience where you wake up the next day and you're all good. It's like an injury that requires time to heal. For days, weeks, and months after the event, I felt the tightness in my chest. With each presentation, meeting, discussion, and work challenge, I sensed that I was walking close to the edge of it happening again. Sometimes, I awoke in the middle of the night before a big meeting or presentation, my heart racing and covered in sweat.

I questioned my path forward. I was more than capable as an individual contributor. Perhaps I could focus on quietly doing my work. I could give up some management responsibilities, speaking opportunities, and rapid career growth. Instead, I could remain in places where I was more comfortable. I could still have success, just on different terms.

While contemplating the options, I always knew that remaining in my comfort zone would lead to regret. The underdog in me didn't want to hear about the compromises I could make. But it wasn't just a matter of "choosing the harder path." If I couldn't get past this struggle, which was only intensifying, my body had already informed me that it wasn't coming along for the ride.

***

Let's fast forward almost ten years to the writing of this book. I never had a second panic attack. I no longer have moments where a feeling of doom is looming over my consciousness. I don't wake up in the middle of the night with my heart racing. The stress and anxiety aren't building momentum with a certainty that threatens to overtake me. I'm no longer at the wheel of a semi-truck careening down a mountain road with no brakes.

I feel the opposite. I feel stronger with each day, month, and year that passes. I can sit down with people one-on-one, I can lead meetings, and I can deliver presentations to executives without simultaneously waging an inner war against waves of anxiety. In my personal life, I can step forward as the best man at my friend's wedding, toasting him and his wife in front of hundreds of guests with no notes. As a father of three amazing kids and husband to an incredible wife, I can take control of a demanding work schedule to show up fully present in the big moments and, more importantly, the small ones each day. I can connect purpose with how I spend my time, focusing on the present instead of worrying about the past or future.

When I inevitably veer off course and the stress and anxiety seep in, I have a process for stopping the momentum and getting back on track. I have learned how to go past treating the symptoms of anxiety to address the source. Doing so hasn't required medications, substances, or even innocuous stimulants. While the answer isn't a light switch and requires hard work and discipline, it's a solution within your reach. Let's dive in.

Chapter Two

The Source of Anxiety & The Most Powerful Thought

Before we can solve our anxiety problem, we first need to understand the factors that conspire to produce it. We'll build this understanding in three parts: 1) we'll define our anxiety; 2) we'll explore how anxiety forms in the brain; and 3) we'll identify the thoughts that trigger the anxiety response. Stick with me as we establish this foundation because you'll get your answer to anxiety's source in this chapter, plus the key to its defeat.

1: Defining Anxiety

I've been using the terms stress and anxiety without distinction, but now it will be helpful to separate the two. Stress is an emotional tension triggered by a challenge or stressor. This tension results in different responses, both physical and mental.

Physically, our blood pressure may rise, our muscles may tense, or we might start sweating. Not all stress is bad; it's often beneficial, leading to gains in performance, focus, and enjoyment. Psychologists refer to the "good stress" as "eustress" and the "bad stress" as "distress." The difference between "good stress" and "bad stress" is frequently based on how we perceive the stressor and whether it was introduced by choice or involuntarily thrust upon us. Careening down the track of a rollercoaster will elicit a stress response but also a thrill, excitement, and joy. If instead of a rollercoaster ride, we're driving in a snowstorm and begin sliding down the icy street, the physical sensation may mirror the rollercoaster experience. However, we go from healthy stress to panic as we lose control.[1]

Bad stress and anxiety share the same range of mental and physical responses. The difference between the two is time and place. Anxiety begins with distress, but then it continues past the point of the stressor; we're through the challenge, yet the feeling stays with us. Or, the stress-inducing event is in the future, say a month away, yet we experience stressful feelings in each of the 30 days leading up to the occasion. Stress (or "distress") and anxiety can be likened to the difference between sadness and depression. Stress is like sadness. It's a feeling tied to what's happening in the present. There's a trigger that causes your stress response, but it doesn't persist. When you're through the challenge, the stress leaves with it. Anxiety, on the other hand, is like depression. It lingers with us, often long past the event that served as the trigger or well in advance of it.[2]

Returning to the example of driving on the winter road, if an experienced winter driver is at the wheel, practiced in dealing with icy conditions, they can feel in control of the situation. They benefit from the heightened focus and mental sharpness their stress is delivering. The car may still be sliding, but they haven't lost the *belief* that they are in control.

Loss of control is what produces negative stress and, if that feeling persists, will lead to worry and anxiety. We worry about a presentation because we can't control how others will perceive it; we worry about the health of a loved one leading up to a medical diagnosis; we worry about them after the diagnosis comes in, as we still can't alter it; we worry about the inability to get pregnant; when we get pregnant, we worry about taking care of the baby; when the baby is born, we worry about their eating, their sleeping, their exposure to germs; we worry about our financial health when our income source is insufficient or in question; we worry about our relationship health, as we only control one side of the connection; we worry that the weather will ruin our vacation; we worry *on* vacation about the work that's piling up as we're away.

Negative stress that lingered and grew into anxiety, is what ultimately led to my panic attack. Others will have different reactions or symptoms that might include exhaustion, physical pain, or problems with digestion. Anxiety can produce feelings of sadness, hopelessness, and depression. It can make you more susceptible to sickness. This book focuses on the negative stress or distress that leads to worry and anxiety. The kind characterized by a loss of control. The stress that we didn't willingly choose but that was involuntarily introduced into our system.

We've now defined the problem, but what's the *cause* of the problem? To understand the driver of anxiety, let's now explore how different processes play out in the brain to produce it.

2: The Role of the Brain

To fulfill our purpose, we can stay at a relatively high level. I'll describe the parts of the brain in broad groupings rather than explore all the discrete regions and their associated functions. It's enough to establish that different brain parts play different roles. These separate brain regions also develop in various life stages, both inside and outside the womb. The two parts of the brain we'll consider are the "emotional brain" (with particular emphasis on the amygdala) and the neocortex or "thinking" or "rational brain." The neocortex is the largest part of the cerebral cortex, the brain's outermost region. This "smart" part of our brain separates us from animals and gives us the capacity for critical thinking. The cortex parts of our brain take the longest to fully develop, with the maturity of some regions continuing through our mid-20s.[3,4,5,6]

The fact that we can add significant value to companies through no more than thinking, forming those thoughts into words, or conveying those thoughts with computer clicks or button presses is a reality made possible by the neocortex. The explosion of what management guru Peter Drucker coined as "knowledge workers" didn't happen until after the second industrial revolution at the turn of the 20th century.[7] However, society has had knowledge workers for centuries. The Romans are famous for their philosophers and senators, whose societal function was to think and effectively communicate those thoughts to others. That's not much different than today when rational thought is the basis of work for me and millions of other knowledge workers. The effectiveness with which we complete that work depends on the proper functioning of the neocortex.

If the neocortex separates us from animals, the emotional brain and other lower brain regions (those sitting "below" the cerebral cortex) bind us to them. These regions, which include the brain stem, the amygdala, and the limbic system, I'll collectively refer to as the "lizard brain," as these are more primitive parts of the brain, with functions and purposes overlapping with the brains of animals. While rational thought comes from the neocortex, the lizard brain generates much of our emotions. The lizard brain is also responsible for many of our instincts and pre-programmed knowledge.

Have you ever considered how babies come out of the womb with the innate understanding to perform different tasks? No one had to teach them how to take their first breath. If we did, I wouldn't have three kids now, as I haven't been able to train any of them to make their breakfast after eight years of trying. Having only a few seconds to teach a newborn how to breathe would undoubtedly bring about their demise. Thank God for the lizard brain. More fascinating than breathing, no one had to sit down and explain that they suddenly needed to eat to survive. "Hey, that cord to your stomach we were feeding you through? Yeah, we cut that off. From now on, put the food in your mouth and it will end up in the same place."

The lizard brain, particularly the amygdala, has other pre-programming to protect us from danger. The amygdala is associated with the emotion of fear and is responsible for the body's "fight-or-flight" reaction, or what is sometimes referred to as "fight, flight, or freeze." This reaction is essential for survival. Our ancestors depended on it, as humans were the prey of larger, stronger, and faster carnivores. Today, it plays the same vital function; that function just shows up in different ways. While we're [hopefully] less likely to be chased down by a tiger as we take a morning walk, there might be a car that unexpectedly comes around the corner on our stroll, which we need to act instantly to avoid. Our lizard brain helps us jump out of the way just in time.

Comparing the parts of the brain with athletes, the lizard brain is a pressure player. It has to come through in the clutch. It needs to work and to work fast. If it doesn't, we don't survive. Knowing it's a pressure player, it's also a bit of a diva. When stress ratchets up, it needs all our resources; in fact, it demands them. As a general in battle, it deploys our physical resources to where they're needed most. Blood is sent rushing to our arms and legs so we can react instantly. Our muscles are primed. Our focus is sharpened.

Yet, we have a finite set of resources. The lizard brain is like a plane's captain entering inclement weather. It tells its copilot, the neocortex, "I'm taking the controls as we enter the storm. I'll let you back into the picture when the seat belt sign is off, and we emerge into clear skies." As we process information from the "bottom up," that information is often withheld from the neocortex at the upper level, temporarily disabling our ability to exercise rational and critical thinking. This emergency lockdown orchestrated by the lizard brain is called the "amygdala hijack."

While we may have situations of extreme panic, like the car careening out of control or delivering a big presentation and freezing up on stage, this process of fear and response orchestrated by the lizard brain and amygdala, doesn't always result in all-out panic or fight-or-flight. My panic attack was the peak event, but I had years of nagging anxiety that sat in the back of my mind leading up to it. The lizard brain was processing the signals, assessing the severity, and responding in kind to different degrees of intensity. Anxiety manifests through these dynamics. We have a lower-level feeling of fear that lingers despite the lack of an immediate stressor. The lizard brain picks up on those worried feelings and starts to jump in, triggering the rise in heart rate, rapid breathing, and the tensing of our muscles. In this way, the lizard brain can *partially* hijack our consciousness, in addition to pulling off a complete heist. We're still able to think, just not as well. Our rational judgment is there, but it's clouded or less responsive.

The fight-or-flight reaction is essential if we're hiking in the woods and unexpectedly encounter a bear, but there are many situations when the stress response delivered by our lizard brain is not only unnecessary, it's counterproductive. Standing in front of a conference table on a Tuesday, we do *not* need to worry about a car speeding through the room and taking us down. And we certainly don't need to worry that the tiger from earlier has figured out how to access our office building and is now roaming the hallways. What we need in that conference room is for our neocortex to be at the controls, operating at peak capacity. Ideally, there would be a way to signal to the lizard brain, "False alarm, you think I'm about to be killed, but I'm just in a status meeting and feeling anxious that my boss will ask about something I don't have a great answer to. Please stop sending all the blood away from my head so I can think for a moment!"

Unfortunately, that off button doesn't exist. Our brains operate more like an aristocracy than a meritocracy. Although the neocortex is better suited to deal with anxiety outbreaks, it has to defer to the lizard brain. For the neocortex to get a well-deserved promotion, the lizard brain has to step aside, which will not happen. And honestly, we don't want to banish it entirely because it's likely to save our lives. We want our lizard brain to do a better job of staying in its lane, jumping into action when it's required. The challenge is that the lizard brain operates based on automation that we can't consciously control.

Though these situations play out on a spectrum ranging from utter panic to mild discomfort, there's a common thread here. In all these situations, there's a perception of danger to varying degrees. A belief that we're not safe. An assessment that we've lost control and are heading to an outcome that is not good. We can't consciously control or "turn off" the lizard brain's stress response; however, that common thread is the key to the trigger that initiates our lizard brain's automation process. We're now ready for the final foundational piece found in our thoughts.

3: The Power in Our Thoughts

CBT, or cognitive behavioral therapy, is a psychotherapy approach underpinned by the principle that our thoughts, feelings, attitudes, emotions, and actions are interconnected. I like the simplified construct that our thoughts drive our feelings, which, in turn, drive our actions. People undergoing cognitive behavioral therapy or CBT first seek to recognize and understand the thoughts and feelings contributing to their actions. Then, they engage in various exercises to correct unhelpful thought patterns and carry those approaches through to the behavior they desire.[8]

I find inspiration in different places. I heard an interview with Tom Brady, the all-time great former quarterback of the New England Patriots and Tampa Bay Buccaneers. Brady was discussing the importance of accountability. He described how we always have a choice before we act.[9] Even if we have an impulse to do something harmful, like react to someone with anger or say something unkind, there is always a moment before the action where we make the choice. Do we follow through with our impulse and act the wrong way? Or, in that split second, do we choose to pivot and take the right course, regardless of our feelings? That observation resonated with me, and I tried to apply it.

One area where I've struggled is getting my kids ready for bed. I wake up in the morning with strength and resolve. I commit to being fully present with them during the day. I tell myself I won't let my anxiety that I need to get to work impact the moments

I have with them before they go to school. I'm excited to enjoy activities with them that make them happy. But by the end of the day, I'm physically tired and, even more so, emotionally worn down. My reserves, replenished from sleep the night before, are running low. I'm ready for them to get to bed and to have some time for myself or with my wife. I'm so close to the finish line, but then it happens. They start splashing me in the face with water while I try and finish their bath. Or my boys conclude they both must hold the same individual Lego piece in their possession, among the sea of 10,000+ Legos we have, and a war breaks out. Or my daughter decides there will be hell to pay unless she can eat a cookie after I've just brushed her teeth. And despite all the good work I've put in through the day, I lose it. I yell at them to *stop* or that the answer is "no!" It happens in an instant, and I immediately regret it. I was so strong through the day, but now, a few seconds of losing control resulted in sending my kids to bed with them upset, feeling like I've been mean, while I'm feeling disappointed in myself.

Why couldn't I be like Tom Brady and, when I felt the impulse to yell, choose instead to speak calmly and finish the day strong? I was so close. All I had to do was hold out for a few more minutes, and the day would be a success, but I blew it. I came to realize that I am not strong enough to choose the right action when that action conflicts with my feelings. Maybe I can do it once or twice, but it's game over by the 8th time that bathwater splashes in my face.

While the field of CBT originated in the 1960s and '70s, this observation that we can't just choose to take the right actions in opposition to our feelings dates back to biblical times. In the

Bible's New Testament, Paul, an apostle of Jesus, wrote in his letter to the Romans, "For I do not understand my own actions. For I do not do what I want, but I do the very thing I hate... For I have the desire to do what is right, but not the ability to carry it out. For I do not do the good I want, but the evil I do not want is what I keep on doing."[10] Paul concluded that the sin living in him was the source of his negative actions. I believe what Paul categorized as his sin was actually his negative thought patterns. He found that these negative thoughts and feelings led to choices that he recognized were harmful but could not be overcome through sheer force of will. If you don't know the story of the Apostle Paul, he was repeatedly beaten, imprisoned, faced calamity, and was ultimately killed for his faith. Paul was not mentally weak, yet he admits to often not being strong enough to follow through on his good intentions when they conflicted with his internal state.

I can relate to Paul. I am not strong enough to choose the right action when it conflicts with my feelings. Going further, I am not in control of my feelings. My feelings are what they are. If I'm angry, I can't flip the switch and turn anger into joy. We cannot alter our feelings because our irrational lizard brain dictates them, just as it directs our stress response. The lizard brain isn't interested in logic and has no off button. But something dictates the feelings and reactions the lizard brain generates, which we can control: our thoughts.

We gain great power in recognizing that our thoughts are malleable and can be deployed to achieve our desired outcomes. In his classic book, *As a Man Thinketh*, author James Allen states, "A man's mind may be likened to a garden, which may be intelligently cultivated or allowed to run wild; but whether cultivated or neglected, it must, and will, bring forth. If no useful seeds are put into it, then an abundance of useless weed seeds will fall therein, and will continue to produce their kind."[11] It's the message of reaping what we sow. Our mind will generate thoughts whether we like it or not. We will yield good outcomes if we plant good seeds through positive thinking. If we plant seeds of negativity, our outcomes will be negative. And even if we don't plant *any* seeds through an intentional process, our subconscious will introduce thoughts on its own. For those struggling with anxiety, the anxious feelings demonstrate that our unconscious is sowing seeds of negativity.

Thinking alone does not physically manifest anything, yet our thoughts fuel the fire of our actions. Close to 2,000 years ago, Marcus Aurelius, the Roman emperor and philosopher, stated, "Our life is what our thoughts make it," and "The happiness of your life depends on the quality of your thoughts."[12] Both James Allen and Marcus Aurelius discovered the powerful truth about the connection between our thoughts and actions long before the founding of CBT as a psychological discipline.

Do you want to overcome anxiety at work? Do you want a home life characterized by love and presence rather than stress? The timeless truth is that those outcomes are within reach when we start with the right thoughts. Instead of focusing on correcting our actions, we shape our thoughts, reinforce them, and then allow the natural outflow of those thoughts into our feelings and actions.

Anxiety's Source Thought

We've established that our harmful stress, which turns to anxiety, results from a perception of danger. The lizard brain picks up on the signal that we're in trouble. It acts by initiating our stress response to a level corresponding to the magnitude of the threat. We want it to act when we're in real danger, but our harmful stress and anxiety coincide with situations when the response is not warranted, like when we're in that conference room feeling anxious. We want to turn it off. So, how do we stop the lizard brain's response? We need to eliminate the perception of danger and the associated feeling of fear. We can successfully remove the feeling by addressing the source thought.

What I realized is that in every situation when I've felt anxiety at work or home, the underlying thought is always the same, "I don't want to be here." When I was about to give a presentation at work, I was thinking, "I can't wait for this to be over." Once completed, I had some good feelings - including accomplishment and satisfaction in a job well done - but those feelings accompanied relief that I was through the uncomfortable situation where I perceived danger.

At VMware, as the anxiety started to creep into more and more interactions, including just sitting across the table from someone having a conversation, the unfortunate reality was the same: I didn't want to be there. It wasn't that I didn't like the people I worked with - I liked most of them quite a bit - but my anxiety had spread to a broad set of interactions, brought about by an underlying thought that accompanied the feeling of danger and acted as its catalyst. The fear of "I'll be exposed" was becoming present in one-on-one settings and group interactions.

It wasn't only anxiety where that thought was present. It took more introspection, but I realized that in the more momentary occurrences of stress, the kind that leads to anxiety if allowed to persist, the same thought was there. For example, the bedtime struggle with my kids wasn't anxiety; that was temporary stress. In those moments, as the bathwater poured onto the floor, or the kids' emotions exploded into tantrums, or the battle to brush their teeth escalated, I had the same thought: I didn't want to be there. I wanted to be done. Unwinding. Sitting downstairs. In that situation, I obviously didn't consciously think I was in danger. Still, with an underlying thought of "I don't want to be here," my mind interpreted the situation the same way it would interpret any other threat, initiating my stress response as a reaction to what it *perceived* was a threat.

What about those other examples of anxiety we covered earlier? Surely, there are different source thoughts in some of those circumstances, like our worry about the health of a loved one, our apprehension about a relationship, or our financial anxiety. Yet in these cases as well, we're sensing danger (or our subconscious is interpreting it as such), and our lizard brain is initiating an impulse to distance ourselves from the source of the perceived threat.

If you think about it, that's a hard reality. The premise is easy to accept if we're talking about giving a presentation – you know you don't want to be *there* – but does that also imply that we "don't want to be there" when we're anxious about a loved one's illness? You might think that you wouldn't want to be anywhere else and that claiming otherwise is insulting. And you'd be right, at least from the perspective of your conscious thoughts and rational brain.

However, there are competing thoughts from your subconscious. They are initiated by your lizard brain, recognizing the danger you perceive and trying to protect you from it. You will fight against it, and that cognitive struggle is a big piece of the anxiety that we'll explore in greater depth. The desire to be there for your loved one is rock solid, but the "I don't want to be here" thought is there as well. And upon reflection, who would *want* to be in a situation with a sick loved one? Of course you don't *want* to have that experience. Yet if you allow that thought to persist in your subconscious at each moment, that continual thought of not wanting to have that experience is what will produce your anxiety. Now, a sick loved one is obviously not a good situation. Seeking to remove our anxiety in such a circumstance doesn't mean we can't have other feelings at the same time. For instance, the feelings of sadness may be profound, but that sadness does not have to be accompanied by anxiety.

To clarify, the source thought may not always be *exactly*, "I don't want to be here." But it will be some variation of an "I don't want to" thought. "I don't want to do this or do that." "I don't want to be here or be there." "I don't want this to be my reality or to have had this experience." The dissonance we feel between what is facing us and what we want is what leads to our anxiety. As we'll explore further, "I don't want to be here" is the most harmful manifestation of these thoughts.

If the underlying thought in all our anxious situations is "I don't want to be here" (or "there" or to do "that"), then it's not the lizard brain that's the problem. The lizard brain seeks to give us exactly what we really want, even desires we're either not consciously aware of or are unwilling to admit. In this way, the lizard brain aligns our feelings and actions with our underlying thoughts. As it turns out, our rational brain may be the real source of our angst. If we sense danger and want to avoid it, our loyal friend, the amygdala, is more than happy to oblige. It attempts to get us out of the uncomfortable situation, like a school buddy pulling the fire alarm to free us from detention.

Conversely, our rational brain essentially holds us against our underlying will. It reasons, "You've got to give this presentation because it's really important." "You committed, and now you need to follow through." "It's your job, for crying out loud. You *have* to do this." Or at home, as we waver when facing bedtime duties with our kids, our rational brain tells us, "The kids aren't going to brush their teeth and turn out the lights on their own, so just get it done as fast as possible." In these cases, the rational arguments formed in the neocortex fight against our base thoughts. The fight-or-flight impulse, and even our anxiety, turn out not to be the enemy that we need to find an "off button" for. Our enemy is the "I don't want to be here" thought itself, with the problem being that we often don't recognize this thought for the unwelcome guest that it is.

I love the Adam Sandler movie *Click*. It's one of those movies you think will be brainless, but it surprisingly leaves you reflecting on your life. In the film, Adam Sandler plays a husband and father to a young and adoring family. Sandler is struggling, though. Finances are tight, and he's long overdue for a promotion at work, which he believes will make life a lot easier. During a visit to the retailer Bed, Bath, and Beyond, Sandler receives a universal remote control with the power to direct not just his electronics but also his life. In particular, it allows him to fast forward through unpleasant daily events. Boring conversation? Fast forward through it. Tedious chore? Fast forward through it. Uncomfortable emotion? Fast forward through it.

The remote also has a special feature that automatically learns his habits and acts on his behalf. As Sandler uses the remote to avoid and control unpleasant circumstances at work, his path to promotion and financial success accelerates. Yet, as he's operating on "autopilot" during the fast forwarding, he neglects his wife and kids, who were the original motivation for the financial advancement. *(Side note: this movie from 2006 already predicted the negative implications of AI).* He eventually speeds forward years into the future, wealthy and successful (though comically overweight), but he loses his family in the process. Fortunately, the experience with the magic remote was all just a dream. As he wakes, he's left with the lesson to not fast forward through life, even the difficult moments.[13]

If the negative thought driving our anxiety is "I don't want to be here," we are also guilty of the same pitfall of fast-forwarding through life. Sure, many situations might present a challenge, but do we *really* want to skip over every challenging experience at work or home? I see my kids changing daily at home and know that each moment is a blessing. I don't want to look up one day and realize I let their childhood pass me by. At work, my goal is continual growth, not just in terms of career progression but professional and personal development. I want to finish each day stronger than I started, with more knowledge, skills, experience, and wisdom. Growth can't happen when sitting in a comfort zone, so these stress-inducing situations are necessary to progress. There is a different lens from which to view these interactions. That alternative perspective also does not require lying to yourself to replace the "I don't want to be here" thought. The key is to replace it with a thought that you *do* believe.

Identifying the harmful underlying thought is a critical part of the process, but it's only half of the equation. Our brains won't operate with a blank slate. Go ahead and give it a try. Think about nothing for a minute... How is that working out? We can't just work to remove the harmful thought and leave nothing in its place. The brain will implement a displacement process and stick some other thought there. Letting thoughts enter our minds without intention is what got us into trouble with anxiety in the first place. Instead of allowing the brain to fill the space with another thought that may be harmful or even just non-helpful, we need to actively replace that thought of "I don't want to be here" with a value-adding alternative.

The Most Powerful Thought

One of the exercises commonly employed through CBT treatments is a technique called "opposite action."[14] It means just what you'd think. When you have an impulse to do something harmful or problematic, before you act, come prepared with an action that's the polar opposite and choose to do that instead. For instance, if you struggle with frustration towards your coworkers, often leading to tense interactions, decide in advance that you will compliment them the next time you are triggered. Your impulse will be confrontation, but your action will be to praise. As it's challenging to come up with compliments in the face of frustration, you'll identify areas of admiration in advance that are genuine and that you can deploy when needed.

This exercise is one of the implementations of CBT that I find problematic. If our thoughts, feelings, and actions are all connected, asking people to act the opposite of how they feel is, more often than not, a losing proposition, mainly because the lizard brain and the limbic system are responsible for our feelings and emotional reactions. Once you start experiencing a powerful emotion, the pull to act in step with that emotion may be too great to resist.

While "opposite action" can often be a losing battle, we can apply the same concept earlier in the lifecycle to the domain where we have control: our thoughts. Instead of fighting our impulse to run at the point when we feel anxiety or employing a coping mechanism once the anxiety is already with us, our focus can shift to seeding the right thoughts in advance of the challenging situations we're bound to encounter. The practice I'll refer to as "opposite thought" allows us to choose a thought that runs counter to our sense of danger and the fight-or-flight impulse.

So, what's the opposite thought of "I don't want to be here?" You guessed it, "I want to be here." "I want to be in this room, giving this presentation right now." "I want to be participating in this meeting." "I want to be here socializing with my coworkers." "I want to be called on in this session to share my point of view. I'm not here to hide but to be seen and make an impact." And at home: "I want to be here with my kids during the last moments of their day. I will make the time special for them, as it is a special time for me." There is great power in the thought, "I want to be here." You turn from a hostage to a willing and eager participant.

Rather than waiting for your fear-response reaction to play out, take the approach to seed the right thought proactively, priming the desired feelings to be present as you go into a potentially challenging situation. The reframing happens before anxiety has the chance to strike. The concept of "opposite thought" is easy to articulate, but we need to be ready for the challenge in its implementation. If you've struggled with anxiety, the "I don't want to be here" thought has likely been living rent-free in your mind for years. This unwanted thought is embedded and hiding behind many of your suboptimal interactions. Uprooting and replacing a harmful thought is part of a process that takes time and purposeful effort. The cycle from thoughts to feelings to actions can be instantaneous, so once our thinking has gone astray, our feelings have already followed close behind. We must be intentional in cultivating our thoughts, accomplishing this state through planning, activation, and reinforcement.

***

A connected chain leads to our actions. It starts with our thoughts, transfers to our feelings, and is visible through our behaviors. When we experience harmful stress that lingers and becomes anxiety, those feelings follow a perception of danger, whether real or contrived by our subconscious. Behind this process is the thought, "I don't want to be here."

The belief that we're in danger or facing a threat is most apparent when we're in all-out fight-or-flight mode, as the lizard brain hijacks our consciousness, disallowing the function of our "higher" areas of the brain. However, the source thought, "I don't want to be here," is lurking across the broader range of situations where you feel stress and anxiety. This thought and its associated feelings result in experiences that are unpleasant and often regrettable. While our feelings are automatic, and it's hard to act in a way that conflicts with them, we can go one step further back to disrupt the process. By choosing our thoughts, we powerfully shape our mental state and experiences. These thoughts, and in particular, the "I want to be here" thought, hold the key to conquering our stress and anxiety.

Chapter Three

The Process

A common myth is that we only use 10% of our brains. As scientists have studied the brain through imaging technology, they've witnessed activity in all parts of the brain, both waking and sleeping.[1] We may not fully understand each function, but we know it's up to something. *(Side note: I would argue that when my kids watch the TV show SpongeBob SquarePants, they are temporarily stuck in the realm of 10% brain activity, but that's a question requiring further study.)*

While we do use our brains, some scientists estimate that 95% of our brain activity operates at the subconscious or unconscious levels.[2] Go ahead and think, "I want to be here." That's a conscious thought. But right after you've repeated that thought, your mind will likely return to a range of subconscious thinking. As you read this chapter, you're assessing what I'm saying. You're thinking about how it relates to your life and the connection to your personal experiences. Your mind may wander as you think about a meeting you need to attend or an e-mail you need to return. You're thinking about whether you agree or disagree with the content. Does this message align or conflict with your beliefs? You may have thought about your own guilty pleasure shows when I mentioned SpongeBob. You're not *trying* to form those thoughts. They just appear. For every conscious, intentional thought, there will be a collective of more automatic ones.

Fortunately, while most of our thoughts are automatic, that doesn't mean they are inaccessible. They just take reflection to uncover. Have you ever been annoyed with someone and realized that you had an entire argument with them in your head that they weren't even a part of? Imagine this scenario: You took a break at work and returned to find the instant message from your boss, "Can you send me the project proposal as soon as possible?" Your anxiousness spikes as you put aside the left-overs from your lunch. They will ask where you were when they were trying to reach you. When they do, you'll tell them that you worked last weekend and no one cared to bring *that* up, so why are *they* bringing attention to a 30-minute break for lunch? In addition, you started the day at 7 in the morning, when they didn't show up until 8:30. You worked an hour and a half before they even walked in the door!

Suddenly, you realize you're feeling angry towards your boss. Who do they think they are to question your work ethic? But all they asked you for was to send a file. The argument never happened. The claims about your work ethic or availability were a product of your thoughts, not their words. Yet those thoughts led to feelings of anger, which make it hard to have a genuinely positive interaction when you deliver that proposal. While this "argument" may have played out through your subconscious, the good news is that the hypothetical exchange is accessible to your conscious mind. Your thoughts are simply the ongoing dialogue you have with yourself. Even if that conversation happens in the background, you can uncover it with some digging.

Before beginning to work through your thoughts, you need to make space for what should be a daily process. If you don't prioritize intentional reflection and planning, you will repeat the same negative or suboptimal patterns. At work, what do we do after delivering a big presentation? We have a debrief with our team to assess how it went. What went well? What could be improved? Were there questions that we didn't anticipate or have a good answer to? For projects that take several weeks or months to complete, often there will be a "post-mortem" meeting at their conclusion, where the team comes together in a structured way to dig through the project's lifecycle. Did it come in on time and budget? Did it meet the business objectives? Did the team work well together? In cases where the answer is "no" or "not entirely," a discussion is initiated to explore the root causes. In sports, the best players and coaches watch film of their games and analyze each play. What plays were effective and why? When something went wrong, what sequence of events led to it? Was it a failure of the strategy or in the execution of the strategy? In the same way, run back the tape of your past 24 hours. How did you do yesterday? What went well, and what could have gone better?

In his book *Never Finished*, former Navy Seal and elite endurance athlete David Goggins describes his practice of a "morning meeting." A morning meeting doesn't sound particularly special, but the twist is that *he* is the only attendee. Goggins observes that we spend much of our days at work in meetings, often for the benefit of others, but why don't we give that same attention and focus to better ourselves? He carves out time with himself in the morning for reflection on yesterday and planning for the day ahead. Where did he go wrong yesterday? How can he turn that around today? Goggins is a proponent of having hard conversations with yourself, being honest about where you've fallen short, developing a plan to address it, and taking action.[3]

My practice is similar, but my morning meeting is a prayer. Each morning, I wake up, get dressed, and get my running shoes on. I typically listen to an audiobook when I run, but that time in the morning is about getting ready for the day ahead, so I leave all devices behind. I head out for a half-hour jog. As I take my first steps, I begin. I treat prayer like an informal conversation. The dialogue has three parts: 1) thanksgiving, 2) reflection and root cause analysis, and 3) planning for the day. Whether it's a prayer or a meeting with yourself, the structure of that conversation can be the same.

I start with thanksgiving. Thanksgiving for being alive, having strength in my body to run, living in a beautiful place, passing by trees, and having a family to share life with. I reflect on the previous day and my gratitude for those experiences. Our perspective is often clearest in the morning. Our anger during yesterday's argument with a loved one has faded. What remains is our appreciation for the relationship and a renewed resolve to show them our love. I thank God for the meaningful people in my life and for the experiences we shared. I reflect on the small moments of joy and fulfillment. Starting from a place of optimism is an essential foundation that prepares us for the challenging work ahead.

Reflection and Root Cause Analysis

After giving thanks, the second stage is to reflect on and analyze the prior day's events to identify the underlying emotional and behavioral drivers. In evaluating our negative experiences, we can discover the undesirable thoughts that shaped them. To root out your negative thoughts, you must start beyond them, assessing your feelings or actions. You have thousands of individual thoughts daily, with most of those operating at the subconscious level. Isolating the harmful ones is a needle-in-a-haystack undertaking. Instead of starting your search for the thought, flip the CBT progression and begin with the action.

What's something you *did* over the past day that you're not proud of, or was a notably negative interaction, or was misaligned with your values? Perhaps it was sending a passive-aggressive e-mail to that boss who "accused you" of being away from your desk for too long. "Hi Sally. If you told me that you needed the proposal yesterday, I could have sent it at 7 a.m., when I was the first person in the office. Here it is, but now we don't have any time for revision." What feeling drove that action? Well, you were angry and feeling defensive that they reached out to you on your lunch break, expecting (or so you thought) an immediate response. What's the core thought driving that feeling of anger? Here is where you have to dig into your subconscious. We know you had the hypothetical argument, which played out in your inner dialogue, but what was the thought or belief that drove the "disagreement?" The thought is that your boss doesn't trust you. That they don't think you're working hard or that they're unlikely to give you the benefit of the doubt. While that sentiment may or may not be accurate, what you do know is that all they asked for was a proposal, yet you responded with a passive-aggressive message.

Taking the approach of "opposite thought," you can work to replace your automatic thoughts with more helpful ones, such as, "My boss has good intentions." "My boss trusts me to manage my time effectively." "My boss values the hard work I put in." This process isn't about fooling yourself, though. Maybe your boss *is* a jerk. In that case, "My boss trusts me" will only ring hollow. But what thought could be true that replaces your negative thoughts, fueling your negative feelings? Perhaps it's, "My boss deserves my respect, and I will show them respect in every interaction." The key is to cultivate these thoughts in advance. Repeat them in your mind. Make a plan to recite them when the wrong thoughts about your boss seep in or the next time you are triggered.

What about stress and anxiety? How do we work through the thoughts that contributed to *those* feelings? After all, stress and anxiety aren't "mistakes" identifiable through negative actions. Think about any times yesterday when an event triggered your stress response. As an example, going through our family credit card expenses can be a stress trigger for me. Growing up, I witnessed financial hardships that I recognize had a lasting impact. These experiences shaped what can often be not just an abundance of caution and frugality but an outright unhealthy relationship with money.

On the other hand, my wife Suzy is more of a normal person when it comes to spending. When she needs something, she gets it, and she does the same with our kids. We have a daughter, so I'm learning about all the hair products required for maintaining long hair. It's often hard for me to appreciate that the $5 industrial-sized tub of shampoo, which lasts me three years, doesn't quite meet the haircare needs of my wife and daughter. With this backdrop in mind, I might look at the credit card statement and see a $100 charge for a shampoo product. A feeling of bewilderment overtakes me. Just then, an Amazon delivery man comes into my view, struggling to balance seven boxes on his way to our front door. The stress response is triggered. Suzy walks by. I know I shouldn't, but I comment sarcastically about the purchases.

Now, there's a healthy way to have a conversation about money, and there's an unhealthy way. Sarcasm would not be high on my "relationship best practices" list. To understand the root cause, I need to examine why I arrived at that unhealthy interaction and be open to the potential that I harbor some negative thoughts driving my unwelcome behavior, ones I may not want to admit. The story I tell myself is that I'm just being responsible, providing for my family, and being a good steward of our resources. What a guy I am, right? But underneath, I've found there are other thoughts. I often have a scarcity mindset about money, believing I don't have enough. Or I might be thinking that Suzy is spending too much or doesn't need what she's getting. The beauty in digging deep and uncovering those thoughts is that I can recognize their lies. I can identify that they are thoughts I don't want to have. And I can correct them.

When we were first dating, I may not have been able to afford $100 shampoo, but if it made her happy, I would gladly invest in an overpriced variety gift basket of soaps. I know that mindset of focusing on her happiness is what I want to maintain, even years into our marriage. I want to take care of her and our kids. The resources we have are there for them, after all. So, I choose my truth and my thoughts to coincide with that truth. Applying the opposite thought technique, I declare the thoughts and mindset I want to have related to money and spending. I seed the thought, "Whatever purchases we make as a family today, they will be my signal to initiate thoughts of pride. Pride that I can help to provide good things for them. I am thankful we have resources that can be used on the people I love." Separately, suppose we need to have a spending or budgeting conversation, as couples often do. In that case, I can initiate the conversation in a healthy, constructive way and without sarcasm.

I may continue to get it wrong, and Suzy may tell you this exact issue drives her crazy today, but I'm not accepting the status quo of "this is just the way that I am." I won't accept the negative thoughts that have burrowed their way into my subconscious. Those thoughts may still take residence in my mind, but they are unwelcome guests I am working to evict. I'm retraining the thoughts that color negative interactions with the people I care about the most. Instead of trying to change everyone around me, I consciously focus on how to change myself through my thoughts. *(Side note: Suzy will insist that the $100 shampoo package included three bottles and that they were on sale for 30% off, so when you really think about it, we actually saved money.)*

That's deconstructing our stress response. Now, what about anxiety? At what points yesterday did the feelings of anxiety persist, even well past a trigger or immediate stressor? Our anxiety comes from our worry about what's transpired in the past or our apprehension about events to come. Think about it. If you admit to feeling anxious to a friend and they ask you what you're anxious about, the answer is never what's happening right now. When we're fully present in the moment, we don't allow anxiety to exist. This fact presents a means to help identify the moments when anxiety peaks. How often have you said, "I just need to get through this meeting," "day" or "week?" Those words are a signal of where our anxiety is lurking. We want to "get through" moments rather than experience them. Behind that mentality is the core negative thought, "I don't want to be here."

Leading up to my panic attack, requests to deliver presentations would trigger my stress response and then manifest as anxiety as the feelings lingered. The presentation could be tomorrow, next week, or not for another month. While I answered "yes" outwardly, I had mentally transported myself to the future. The problem was that I was transporting only my current state instead of envisioning the future well-prepared version of me. Was I prepared to deliver the presentation that was a month away right there at that moment? No, and potentially for a variety of reasons. Of course, the top reason is that I hadn't prepared yet. How could I when I just found out about it right now? In addition, the presentation didn't exist yet, and perhaps the project in question was still in progress.

If I was going to project myself into the future, I needed to envision the future me who was well-prepared. The one who finished the project, carefully assembled the presentation, and spent hours preparing and practicing the delivery. The immediate thoughts running through me were, "I'm not ready to do this." "I'm going to embarrass myself." "Surely, someone else is better qualified." I needed an opposite thought. I began to prepare the thoughts I wanted to have. Thoughts like, "They're asking me because I am the best person for the job." "I have a process that ensures I will be prepared when the time comes to perform." "I may not be ready right now, but I will be when it matters."

The more troubling experience was when my anxiety symptoms began appearing even in informal meetings and one-on-one discussions. What was going on, and why was it getting worse? I needed to follow the thread of my anxious symptoms back to the thoughts that produced them. Success can be a powerful driver in building confidence, but there's a flip side to success. The higher you climb, the further there is to fall. Sometimes it's easy to perform when the expectations are low. We see this dynamic in professional sports all the time.

Alex Rodriguez was an up-and-coming star on the Seattle Mariners professional baseball team in the mid-to-late 1990s. While he came into the Major Leagues as a highly touted prospect, he began exhibiting performance in line with the best players in the game immediately during his first full season in the starting lineup. Rodriguez was one of the most popular players in baseball during his time with the Mariners, where, at his financial peak, he made no more than $3 million per season with the team. In 2001, his contract ended, and he entered the free agent market.

Rodriguez left the Mariners to sign the largest contract in baseball history with the Texas Rangers, who agreed to pay him

$252 million over a 10-year contract term. Until then, baseball contracts were measured by the millions they generated, with only a handful of players having eclipsed the $100 million threshold. Rodriguez's contract completely reshaped the narrative: a baseball player was now making a quarter of a *billion* dollars. His average annual salary had increased tenfold. He went from an overperforming up-and-comer to obscenely overpaid in the eyes of the public. The season before, he was one of the most widely admired players in the game. The very next year, he became the most derided. At his games, fans would throw Monopoly money from the stands and rain down boos when he came up to bat. He had gone from hero to villain simply because of his promotion.

In the small market of Seattle and with a relatively modest salary, Rodriguez could play unburdened. In light of $252 million, the pressure exploded. Rodriguez recounted, "When I arrived in Texas in 2001, I felt an enormous amount of pressure. I felt like I had all the weight of the world on top of me, and I needed to perform and perform at a high level every day."[4] The pressure and weight of expectations overcame Rodriguez, as he later admitted to taking performance-enhancing drugs when he joined the Rangers. While his production remained high, he had cheated to attain it when all he needed was to continue with the level of play he had already established in Seattle. He was suspended an entire season for his steroid use, and his legacy as one of the greatest baseball players in history was tarnished.

If you perform above the expectations for your level, it's a pleasant surprise. But once you get that elevated role, the corner office, or the big salary, heightened expectations come alongside the higher position. Your previous outperformance becomes the new minimum standard. When I thought I had "made it" at VMware, I put myself under more pressure than ever before and began to crack. My underdog mentality established a "prove it" mindset, which drove my work ethic but became a double-edged sword. Painting myself as the "underdog" meant everyone was betting against me, expecting me to fail, and judging my every move. That's why my anxiety responses began to spread to even basic interactions. I was plotting my path to success through the subjective judgments of everyone around me. Why was I suddenly finding it difficult to sit alongside my teammates in a small gathering or even one-on-one discussion? Yes, it was because my subconscious told me I didn't want to be there, but that conclusion didn't come from my feelings about the people I was meeting. I didn't want to be there because I didn't want to be judged and found lacking, and I believed that was exactly what was happening. I had to reverse those thoughts.

To deal with the negative thinking, I could have focused on thoughts that refuted my negativity, such as, "No one needs to validate me. I'm already validated. I *am* capable of living up to the expectations." I tried practicing those affirmations. They were true, but they were also an argument against the negative thoughts I was battling. By arguing against them, I acknowledged their lasting presence. I would continue breathing life into them through this approach, even if I tried to keep them bottled up. What I found more effective was to focus my thoughts on the *purpose* of why I was there.

I planned and repeated my thoughts in advance, "I'm here to make an impact. I'm here to help us make better decisions. I'm here to engage through sharing my opinions and recommendations." The key was focusing on the proper division of responsibilities. Who knows, maybe some of those people *were* judging me, but ultimately that didn't matter. I had no control over whether they would choose to judge or not. That was "their job." My job was to focus on my reason for being there. Focusing on their job put me in a powerless state of anxiety as I awaited an outcome I had no control over.

It took considerable time to overcome both the performance anxiety brought about by the presentations as well as to get past the pressure I was feeling from the more routine interactions. At first, I would have to fight back the negative thoughts each time, countering them with my planned replacement thoughts. I repeated these thoughts during my morning routine, as well as before and often during each exchange. Progress came, though it was gradual. It didn't happen all at once, and there were many examples of taking two steps forward and one step back, but as I persisted, the anxiety continued to fade.

I still felt momentary stress and pressure associated with these interactions, but those feelings no longer stayed with me indefinitely. Now, when someone asked me to deliver a presentation, I didn't have a mini moment of panic. While I may not be ready right then, I knew that wasn't the question I was being asked. I could logically assess the request to determine whether it was an important use of my time, whether I had an adequate opportunity to prepare to the necessary level, and whether I was the right person to fulfill the request. Focusing on those questions gave me a range of options that I could evaluate and answer objectively, rather than letting the irrational anxiety hijack what could otherwise be a dispassionate and objective assessment.

With the routine interactions and meetings with my teammates, I could focus on my purpose for being there. I could rely on what I *did* know instead of worrying about what I didn't. If a gap in my knowledge was "exposed," that was a learning opportunity, not a strike against my competence and qualifications. I kept repeating my replacement thoughts. At first, the negative thoughts had the place of preeminence. They were the incumbent and required displacement. As I persisted in practice and time passed, a shift began. The positive thoughts started showing up first. Eventually, they became the *new* incumbent and were there without me having to conjure them up.

What had happened? And why was I suddenly finding it easier to think the right thoughts? It's because of a process called neuroplasticity.[5] Neurons are the cells in the brain and other locations in the body that send chemical and electrical signals through synapse connections to control our physical and mental processes. When a baby takes her first steps, neurons send signals to her legs to move in a way that propels her forward. Those signals follow a track called a neural pathway. These neural pathways begin like a trek through a dense forest. We have to hack our way through branches, leaves, and bushes to get to our destination. But if we walk the same line daily, a path will eventually form amidst the brush. The initial experience of learning to walk represents not just a significant physical challenge but an enormous cognitive test as well, as the required pathways are not yet cultivated. As the neural pathway for walking is repeated and reinforced, the process of walking gets easier and, after time, requires no conscious thought.

The exercise of shaping your thoughts follows the same process. For ingrained negative thought patterns, your brain has neural pathways established that it wants to take. Introducing opposite positive thoughts pushes your brain to trek through the forest instead of taking a freshly paved walking path. You must focus and demonstrate persistence to establish a trail in that forest terrain. If you keep reinforcing the right thoughts, after some time, that path eventually doesn't feel like you need a machete to hack your way through. You observe that the trail feels familiar as you walk it by habit rather than intention. You notice the old path with the negative thoughts. It looks neglected. The concrete is cracking. Weeds are starting to grow over it. It's still there, but the appeal is gone. You've upgraded to the new path.

With anxiety, the wrong thoughts can be deeply embedded and require persistence to uproot. Often, I repeat a similar dialogue in my morning routine and throughout the day to reinforce the desired thinking. Without variation, I might repeat my replacement thought thousands of times over months. Repetition is required. Initially, you have to drill in those replacement thoughts through conscious intention. Over time, they become embedded in your mind and will appear automatically and unconsciously.

***

Let's return to the morning ritual. As you immerse yourself in the "reflection" phase of your morning dialogue, it's clear that arriving at the root cause of these more significant issues and lasting anxieties takes some serious digging. Time will likely extend beyond what you've allotted in the morning session. Once you commit to diagnosing your feelings and actions to get to their root thoughts, begin taking mental or physical notes as you go through each day. As it happens, note it down. Did your anxiety about a work deliverable cause you to miss out on being present in a small interaction with your spouse or kids? Note it down. Did you notice that your attention started to slip in a one-on-one discussion as your anxious thoughts drifted to an upcoming meeting? Note it down. Did an exchange with your boss cause your heart to race? Note it down. In some of these situations, the cause of the anxiety will be clear, and in others, only the anxious feeling will be evident. That feeling is the starting point for a diagnosis in the latter cases. You work backward from the feeling to the root thought.

For the more significant issues that plague you continually, address those both consciously and unconsciously. For instance, identify a situation where your anxiety is recurrent. Perhaps for you, anxious feelings always surface in the presence of a specific person, during a particular activity, or at a certain time of the day. Once identified, begin contemplating the source of that anxiety. You don't have to sit there in meditative thought for hours. Reflect on what's happening, and then go do something else. Frame the problem and establish the desire to arrive at the root thought. Even if you can't solve it immediately, commit to cracking the code. Your brain will keep working through the day and even as you sleep. As long as you remain driven to answer the question, you may find that the solution comes when you're taking a walk, doing the dishes, or after sleeping on it.

Make Your Plan

Once you've completed yesterday's reflection and root cause analysis, get proactive about the challenges you'll face in the day ahead. This last part of the morning routine is your planning session. As your moments of thanksgiving are the introduction, and reflection and root cause analysis can be spread throughout your day, allocate most of your morning routine to the planning phase.

Treat your morning planning time as you would a planning session at work. Mentally review what you have on your schedule. Identify the situations where you're likely to get tripped up with the wrong thinking. Maybe you tend to struggle immediately after work, bringing the anxieties of your job home with you and laying those on your family. Get your plan ready. Tell yourself, "Before I walk in the door, I will remind myself that I'm about to experience the best part of my day when I get to be with my family. I want to be there with them. Even though I had an intense day at work, I'm leaving those challenges at the office. I'm excited for the evening ahead with my spouse and kids. They will feel through my attitude that I want to be present." Plan those thoughts in the morning and repeat them as you enter the situation.

Where did your reflection time indicate you went wrong yesterday? Maybe you had a sub-optimal interaction with your significant other. They wanted to watch a TV show, while you wanted to watch a movie. Instead of compromising, you ended up retreating to separate rooms and each watching alone. You go to bed with an anxious feeling that your relationship is heading in the wrong direction. The following morning, as you reflect on the exchange, you recognize that the movie you watched alone wasn't worth the lack of connection, not to mention it's available on demand and didn't *have* to be watched last night. You identify your underlying thoughts related to control and realize you've been telling yourself that you are *always* the one to compromise and that you *never* get your way. But what you really want is connection. You choose your replacement thought, "Connection with my significant other is my top priority." You plan that when it's time to sit down after dinner and turn the TV on, that is the thought you'll be repeating. When the situation comes up, you consciously repeat that statement. After a few weeks, you're surprised to find that you no longer care *what* you're watching; what matters is *who* you're watching with. You've started to believe the thought, and the thought is transitioning from conscious to subconscious.

Turning to the workday, do you have a crazy meeting schedule today? How will you feel when you're going back-to-back in meetings as e-mails pile up and instant messages roll in? What about your presentation or the group discussion you're leading? Do you feel ready for it, or are you approaching it with apprehension? Consider all your upcoming engagements. If there are any you don't need to be a part of, opt-out (more on that later), but for any activity you're sticking with, go in armed with your planned thoughts.

Pay particular attention to anything on your calendar you're looking to "get through" or "survive." Reframing is a valuable tool to flip your mental narrative on these activities. I've often been in meetings where I'm supposed to be the expert on a particular subject, yet I'm surrounded by highly capable people who I suspect know just as much or more about the topic than I do. The imposter syndrome thoughts begin to creep in. My subconscious tells me, "You'd better get out of this meeting quickly before being exposed." With each question that's posed, I'm simultaneously watching the clock. "OK, I got through that one. Fifteen minutes left. Probably only a few more questions, and I'll have survived." That low-level fight-or-flight response is kicking in, limiting my mental capacity for critical thinking when I need it the most.

When we find ourselves in these situations, we've covered how focusing our thoughts on our purpose is a powerful tool to avoid getting sucked into a fear of exposure. But say that something *does* come up that you have no answer to. What's your plan for *that*? Yes, it starts with a mindset of, "I want to be here," but *why* do we want to be there? Learning is part of our motivation for being among a group of intelligent people. When faced with a question we don't have the answer to, we can perceive that gap in knowledge as a failure, flaw, or deficiency. Alternatively, we can reframe the knowledge gap as a learning opportunity. A growth mindset means that if we don't know something or aren't good at something today, we believe we can gain the requisite knowledge or skills necessary for proficiency through our effort.[6]

If we're learning something new every day, then the version of ourselves now will be stronger than the version of us last year, last month, or even yesterday. Being faced with a difficult question we don't know the answer to can be flipped from problem to opportunity. We want to be in that moment to gain the knowledge that will help us to show up better the next time. If you bluff your way through a situation, you leave with the same lack of understanding you had before. Feeling inadequate or embarrassed about not knowing something impacts your confidence and how you present yourself to others. Suppose we instead own what we don't know and seek education. In that case, we'll leave the encounter stronger, having gained new skills, knowledge, or experience, while still coming across as confident and assertive.

Identify if you're hesitantly approaching something on your calendar, thinking you just need to "get through it." Consider new purposes for being there as options for reframing. Perhaps you're in that meeting to contribute, but when something comes up you don't have the answer to, you're there to learn as well. Maybe you need to have a difficult conversation with a teammate, but it could be reframed as an opportunity to help them instead. Or perhaps you have yet another status meeting where you're typically a passive consumer, but you can reframe your role as an active participant.

In the early implementation of my morning routine, I was naming my mistakes from the day before, but I was missing the planning stage, where I would prepare the right thoughts and reinforce them throughout the day. The result? Frustration. I continued to repeat the same mistakes. Recognizing those missteps and committing myself to doing better was not enough. It wasn't until I began intentionally planning my thoughts that I saw progress. That progress wasn't because I was suppressing my actions. I no longer wanted to act in the old ways because my thoughts had shifted. I continued planning, repetition, and reinforcement, allowing the neural pathways to build until my subconscious was ready to take over.

Your planned thoughts can take innumerable forms tailored to your unique circumstances, but you need a default thought as part of your plan. Your anxiety has its default thought. When it creeps in as your subconscious senses danger, your mind tells you, "I don't want to be here." Be ready with your default, "I want to be here." Remember that being present in the moment and anxiety cannot coexist. When you are anxious, your mind is off worrying about the future or ruminating on the past. You are focusing on the present moment by reminding yourself that you want to be here.

What are those moments that are likely to produce anxious thoughts? Maybe you feel anxiety right before you check your e-mail for the first time in the day. Or perhaps it's right before you walk into a meeting. Or it could be as you see a call coming in from your boss, your apprehension spikes. Recognize that you are choosing to engage in the activity. Nothing is forced on you. You are in control, and you are engaging because you want to.

Your morning routine establishes the plan, but you then need to execute that plan. You have your replacement thoughts ready when the wrong thinking appears, but better yet, be proactive. Don't wait for the negative thoughts to appear before practicing the right ones. As you walk into that meeting, before you check your e-mail, or before that call to your boss, you've already begun repeating your pre-planned thoughts.

***

Commit to a daily practice of 1) thanksgiving, 2) reflection and root cause analysis, and 3) planning for the day. I complete this process each morning as I run, but you can do yours while walking, standing, stretching, or commuting. Note your occurrences of stress and anxiety, as well as other harmful thoughts, as you go through each day. Ask yourself, "What situations was I just trying to 'get through' today?" Pull up your mental or physical list of recent missteps as you begin your morning routine. Where the wrong thoughts have persisted or where lasting anxiety has manifested, leverage repetition to establish new neural pathways that supplant existing ones. Review your schedule and identify the areas where the wrong thoughts will likely appear. Plan the thoughts you'll walk into those situations repeating. Be wary of anxiety's default thought, "I don't want to be here," and always be ready with *your* conscious default, "I want to be here."

Chapter Four

Power in Presence

We are never in the future. We are never in the past. All we have is right now. And where you are is also where you have chosen to be. In whatever way you have decided to spend your present moments, why not realize the full potential of that experience? Our mind has a powerful store of resources we can wield to optimize our experiences and our performance in the present. However, if we are not present, if the anxieties of life and work bring us away to worry about what's ahead or agonize about the past, we sabotage our ability to deliver, engage, and enjoy.

***

George H.W. Bush was the 41st president of the United States, serving one term from 1989 to 1993. Yet Bush wanted to be a two-term president. In the 1992 presidential election, the incumbent Bush faced off against Bill Clinton and Ross Perot. Going into the second debate at the University of Richmond, Virginia, the polls showed a close race between Bush and Clinton, with Bush needing a solid performance to close a slight lead Clinton had developed. This debate featured a unique, town-hall-style format, where the candidates were asked questions from undecided voters present in the audience.

About halfway through the hour-and-a-half debate, a woman named Marisa Hall comes forward to ask a question. But right as she starts to speak, the cameras catch Bush looking at his watch. And he doesn't just glance at his watch. He stands up, lifts his arm to chest-height, adjusts the watch with his opposite hand, and actually takes a step that positions his body away from the questioner. If you freeze the video, you'll see Bush standing with his body facing the audience opposite the questioner, looking down at his watch, while Clinton and Perot sit facing the questioner with their eyes locked on her.

Her question was, "How has the national debt personally affected each of your lives? And if it hasn't, how can you honestly find a cure for the economic problems of the common people if you have no experience in what's ailing them?" Ross Perot answers first, with Bush going second, giving Bush time to plan his response. After Perot finishes, Bush begins his reply, "Well, I think the national debt affects everybody. Obviously, it has a lot to do with interest rates. It has...," but Marisa Hall interjects at this point and clarifies she is asking how the national debt affects Bush *personally*.

Bush then begins to stumble as he starts speaking again. As he realizes he still isn't answering the question, he pushes back on Hall, "Maybe I — get it wrong. Are you suggesting that if somebody has means that the national debt doesn't affect them? I'm not sure I get it. Help me with the question and I'll try and answer it." Marisa Hall clarifies again, this time making a personal connection, "Well, I've had friends that have been laid off from jobs. I know people who cannot afford to pay the mortgage on their homes or their car payment. I have personal problems with the national debt. But how has it affected you? And if you have no experience in it, how can you help us if you don't know what we're feeling?" It should have been clear to Bush that the woman was distressed and was in a community where she felt surrounded by financial hardship. At this point, instead of displaying empathy, Bush makes some strange points about teenage pregnancies and then tells Marisa Hall that it isn't fair to say that just because someone hasn't experienced a particular challenge personally, they can't appreciate what that experience is like.[1]

Clinton is the last to respond. Instead of remaining seated, and in stark contrast to Bush, Clinton walks right up to Marisa Hall. Before answering, he confirms with her, "You know people who have lost their jobs and lost their homes?" Only when she confirms does he begin his answer, "Well, I've been governor of a small state for 12 years. I'll tell you how it's affected me. Every year, Congress and the president sign laws that make us do more things and give us less money to do it with. I see people in my state, middle-class people, their taxes have gone up in Washington and their services have gone down while the wealthy have gotten tax cuts. I have seen what's happened in this last four years. In my state, when people lose their jobs, there's a good chance I'll know them by their names. When a factory closes, I know the people who ran it. When businesses go bankrupt, I know them. And I've been out here for 13 months meeting in meetings just like this ever since October with people like you all over America, people that have lost their jobs, lost their livelihood, lost their health insurance. What I want you to understand is the national debt is not the only cause of that. It is because America has not invested in its people. It is because we've had 12 years of trickle-down economics. We've gone from first to 12th in the world in wages. We've had four years where we've produced no private-sector jobs. Most people are working harder for less money than they were making 10 years ago. It is because we are in the grip of a failed economic theory. And this decision you're about to make better be about what kind of economic theory you want. Not just people saying I want to go fix it, but what are we going to do? What I think we have to do is invest in American jobs, American education, control American health care costs and bring the American people together again."

While Clinton is an incredibly skilled public speaker and empathetic listener, George Bush was also more than capable of delivering in those areas. In fact, in the previous election cycle that won Bush the presidency, Bush and his opponent, Michael Dukakis, were thrown a curveball debate question about how their stance on the death penalty might change if their wives were raped and murdered. Bush answered the shock-value question with a combination of poise and passion. At the same time, Michael Dukakis delivered a robotic response that focused entirely on his well-practiced position on the death penalty while completely ignoring the personal nature of the question.[2] Bush was viewed as relatable, while Dukakis was precisely the opposite.

George Bush *was* highly capable but did not perform to his potential in the debate against Clinton. Why not? Because Bush did not want to be there. Those were his thoughts, which he later admitted in an interview with Jim Lehrer when he described "hating" debates. Recounting the Richmond debate in particular, Bush stated, "Was I glad when the damn thing was over? Yeah, and maybe that's why I was looking at [my watch]. Only ten more minutes of this crap."[3] Referencing the moment he checked his watch, he stated that he "wasn't too conscious of it at all."

Checking his watch and turning away from the questioner were unconscious manifestations of his thoughts, attitude, and feelings about that night. He believed he "had to be there" instead of wanting to be there. His desire to leave was so strong that his watch-checking debacle, which gained notoriety in the press, happened only halfway through the debate rather than within the final ten minutes of the forum, as he mistakenly recalled. He wasn't present. He wasn't listening. He didn't perceive the anguish in the woman's eyes because how could he? He physically wasn't looking at her.

In addition, the question required intentional thought. The backdrop at the time, the early 1990s, was that the country was coming out of a recession and dealing with high levels of unemployment that were peaking during the election cycle. Marisa Hall posed the question and spoke about how people in her community were losing their jobs and couldn't afford to pay their bills. By framing the question around the growing national debt, she concluded that the national debt was the source of her community's economic challenges. That premise was incomplete at best, as the causes of unemployment and the recession were multi-faceted, and a rising national debt often accompanies economic boom times.

Bush should have seen that the real question was about economic struggle and the desire for a leader who was empathetic to that plight. Bush needed to employ critical thinking to recognize the real question and tailor his answer accordingly. Instead, he stuck to the surface issue in his initial response and then became somewhat combative with Hall when she pushed him to speak on the problem from the standpoint of personal experience. He missed the key point because he wasn't present mentally. Clinton, who was fully engaged as Hall spoke, recognized the nuance in the question, demonstrated empathy, and even adeptly informed her that the national debt was not the only cause of the country's economic woes without invalidating her point of view.

When conducting complex tasks that require logical thinking, creativity, or problem-solving, we need the undivided attention of our cerebral cortex, the outer area of the brain that includes the neocortex. Research on multitasking from Kevin Madore, Harvard Ph.D., and Anthony Wagner, Stanford's Deputy Director of the Stanford Wu Tsai Neurosciences Institute, concluded, "When we attempt to multitask, we are usually switching between one task and another. The human brain has evolved to single task."[4] If we try to multitask against the inherent capabilities of our brains, the pair describes that we incur task "switch costs." Two tasks that might take ten minutes if completed one at a time, could take twelve minutes if we attempt to work on both simultaneously. Or, if the time to complete those tasks remains the same, the quality may suffer in the multitasking scenario. When switching between tasks, the brain expends effort to reorient to the new activity, reducing our efficiency.

In considering the research used to support a ban on texting while driving, the Insurance Institute for Highway Safety (IIHS) aggregated the results from 28 independent studies to arrive at their conclusions. Unsurprisingly, they found that when drivers were texting or reading texts, those actions "significantly slowed reaction time, increased lane deviations, and increased the length of time drivers looked away from the roadway."[5] Predicting those outcomes probably didn't require 28 studies to validate because the act of texting means you're physically not looking at the road. More surprisingly, their analysis found that a broader set of cognitive distractions, including even holding a conversation, "can lead to so-called 'inattention blindness' in which drivers fail to comprehend or process information from objects in the roadway even when they are looking at them."

The nuance is that we *can* multitask, but only when using different parts of our brain. For example, we can have deep conversations with a family member, even while we do the dishes simultaneously. The conscious conversation requires the use of our cerebral cortex. Doing the dishes or other behaviors we can perform unconsciously requires using the subcortical parts of the brain located beneath the cerebral cortex. Doing the dishes while engaging in deep conversation is possible only when we've done the dishes so many times that the exercise has become automatic. Had we never done the dishes, we would struggle to focus on that conversation. Go ahead and try to do two things at once that both leverage the critical-thinking parts of your brain.

You could read an article about the political situation in the Middle East while having a meaningful conversation with your significant other. Spoiler alert: that meaningful conversation is about to turn into an argument!

George Bush's act of turning away from the questioner and looking down at his watch occupied his conscious attention. Not because registering the time requires critical thinking but because he was doing more than simply processing the time. When he was thinking, "Ten more minutes of this crap," he was also likely thinking about where he needed to be next. Where he *wanted* to be next. Where he did *not* want to be was in that room, engaging with the undecided voters.

Clinton went on to win the election. He didn't win strictly because of that moment. However, that encounter exemplified Clinton's stronger connection to the needs of the people. He was present and attentive to their needs, while Bush was not. In part of Bush's reply, he stated, "Well, you ought to — you ought to be in the White House for a day and hear what I hear and see what I see and read the mail I read and touch the people that I touch." Bush ended up pushing back on Marisa Hall because *she* didn't know what it was like to be the president when her aim was for the president to understand what it was like to be in her shoes, living in a community personally affected by the ramifications of the recession.

Regardless of our capabilities, our capacity to perform depends on our attention or lack thereof. Have you ever been in a meeting, particularly a virtual one, and started checking your e-mail or answering instant messages simultaneously? What happens when suddenly your name rings out, breaking through your distraction to your conscious attention? You realize that a question is being directed at you. Especially if your boss or other superior is asking the question, you will likely experience a small moment of panic. Your cerebral cortex was occupied, processing the e-mail you were reading or the instant message exchange. You haven't been following the context of the conversation. You're not even sure what the question was. People in this situation might try to fake it by making a comment they believe to be relevant. Or they could ask for clarification. Or they may simply admit they weren't listening. Typically, even if they manage to cobble together a passable response, their lack of attention is evident to the listeners.

I've found that even in one-on-one meetings, my mind can wander. I start thinking about the meeting I have coming up next. I begin reflecting on a particularly challenging problem presented earlier in the day. What's going on in both of those scenarios? I'm physically sitting in that meeting opposite a single other person in real-time. Still, my mind is either in the past, reflecting on events that have already happened, or it's brought me to the future, planning for what's ahead. In neither situation am I fully experiencing what's happening right before me. What a waste of time for both the person I'm meeting and me.

While most people who regularly engage in video meetings are sometimes guilty of this lack of attention, we've all likely experienced this dynamic from the other perspective when our counterpart in the discussion starts to get that glossed-over look in their eyes. You may see their gaze shift or even hear their keyboard going as they respond to an instant message while you're describing the status of a project. As you speak, they may make vague sounds of acknowledgment to present the illusion of listening, but you can see they've mentally left you.

A 2022 study of over 1,000 employees by Showpad found that 76% admit to being more distracted on video calls than in-person meetings.[6] A similar survey of 2,000 American workers by Zippia found that the most common off-task behaviors in virtual meetings include checking e-mails, looking at a cell phone, multitasking on other work, and conducting non-work activities like browsing social media.[7] Multitasking is one consideration, but our focus is also impacted by the mirror of our image staring back at us on video calls. Professor Jeremy Bailenson, Director of Stanford's Virtual Human Interaction Lab, identified the dynamic of seeing ourselves during video calls as one of the principal drivers of "Zoom fatigue" and distraction, as our focus is drawn to our video depiction at the expense of the other participants.[8]

The obvious implication of the rise in remote work is that our physical presence has been cut-off when we switch from in-person engagements to virtual interactions, but our mental presence has also suffered. When we stare at a screen instead of looking someone in the eye, our peripheral vision identifies that we have an unread e-mail or received an instant message. If we begin reading those messages or responding while the meeting is happening, it's not just our attention that's left the conversion, but our critical thinking capabilities. What remains is our background processing mechanisms, listening for keywords, such as our name, as signals to pull us back in. Even if we don't begin reading those incoming messages, being conscious of the notifications themselves can cause our minds to wander as we contemplate who is trying to reach us and consider whether there is something more important calling on our attention.

When I led a customer success team for a technology start-up, we had a bi-weekly meeting with one of the executives at our largest customer. In one of those meetings, as my boss and I joined, the client asked us to wait one minute before starting the discussion. He said that an important message had just come in that he needed to respond to. He would take one minute to respond so that he could be fully present during our discussion. Was I offended that he asked us to wait for a minute or two while he responded? Absolutely not. Instead, I was impressed by his stated value of wanting to be present in our conversation and his acknowledgment that he needed to answer the message to accomplish that state of presence. I would honestly prefer five attentive minutes to thirty distracted ones. I knew that through the rest of the meeting, he was engaged.

Many papers and articles cite the importance of presence. The call to action in these commentaries is typically to remind ourselves to "be present" in the moment. Prompting ourselves to be present can help pull us out of distraction, but those reminders acknowledge that we've already lost our state of presence. Instead of operating in "recovery mode," how can we take a proactive approach and cultivate presence as the default operating characteristic of how we go through our day?

Create an Environment to Foster Presence

Implement a scheduling approach optimized for presence. At work, that means careful management of your meeting calendar. Review all your appointments. Identify the most important ones. Consider, are you prepared? If you aren't and the meeting is of sufficient importance, schedule a time block to get ready. If you don't set aside time to prepare for a key commitment, you'll end up distracted in meetings of lesser importance as your mind wanders and worries about what's ahead. Optimizing your schedule for presence will require prioritization and discernment of the events that are more filler than substance or nonessential. These filler engagements stand in the way of delivering your best in the moments that matter. Have the courage and the discipline to cut them out of your day.

Just as our lack of presence can show up at work as we battle distraction, our reflections about work can follow us home and steal our focus with our family. Before the 2020 COVID-19 pandemic, I would have very little time with my kids during the work week. I'd leave for work before they woke up and return in the evening, only about an hour before their bedtime. Was I working too many hours? Yes, and we'll cover prioritizing our time more in the next chapter. Still, the reality was I had commitments that typically spanned a relatively normal timeframe between 8 a.m. and 5 p.m. Throw in time for commuting, and that doesn't leave a large window for being with young kids, especially when they were still sleeping for close to 12 hours a day *(for non-parents: newborns can sleep up to 20 hours a day and it's typical for kids to sleep up to 12 hours a day through elementary school).*

In 2020, my family moved from the San Francisco Bay Area to Orange County in Southern California. Most office workers were forced into remote work in 2020 due to the pandemic, but my move made the shift to remote work permanent. Among the many benefits? My commute to the corporate office became a trek between my upstairs bedroom and downstairs home office. I could see my kids when they woke up, help get them breakfast, and take them to school. At the time, our pre-school was right around the corner, within a half mile. I would walk or jog my boys in a stroller, drop them off, and return to work. When they started elementary school, I would drive them there as well. I wanted to do these drop-offs and spend this time with them in the morning.

Yet, time after time, my morning interactions with them were colored by stress and anxiety. My meetings often started before their drop-off time and resumed immediately after. I didn't leave much buffer. I was rushing from one meeting to the drop-off and rushing back again. I would often be half-listening to a meeting while completing the process of taking them to school. The lack of boundaries in my schedule allowed anxiety and stress to wash over me and permeate my interactions with my kids.

As parents know, getting young kids to listen, get out the door, and adhere to a tight schedule is probably more daunting than any challenge you'll take on at work. I was physically present, but my mind was off worrying about what would come. The most heartbreaking implication is that my stress was translating to them. As I hurried them along and my frustration grew, they would become upset. Too often, I dropped them off, knowing I had contributed to their feelings of distress to begin their day.

And now the classroom doors were shut, they were gone, and those priceless morning moments had passed me by. A feeling of regret came over me that I had missed another opportunity. As I returned to my desk and entered the meeting that was the source of my anxiety, being there didn't feel quite as urgent as my anxious thoughts had led me to believe a few minutes before.

To break out of this cycle, I had to manage my time more effectively and with greater discretion. Sandwiching that morning time with my kids between two meetings did not provide sufficient space to accomplish my goal. I hoped for meaningful moments when I had budgeted for a mad dash. I had to change my schedule and protect blocks of time that were not open to non-essential meetings. If I needed to prepare for a meeting scheduled immediately after drop-off, I needed to complete that preparation the day before.

Creating the right environment is an essential foundation for realizing our ambitions. Once I had established the necessary boundaries, the most crucial step to achieving presence was intentionally shifting my thoughts as I entered that morning routine with my kids. While I knew I genuinely wanted to be with them, my thoughts asserted a different reality. I thought I needed to get back to work as quickly as possible; that I needed to be highly efficient in that time with my kids to not get off track; and that *they* needed to listen to *my* instructions, or they would negatively impact *my* workday. What it boiled down to is that while my value was to be present at that time, my thoughts all reinforced a false premise of "I don't want to be here." I had to admit that reality to myself. If I wanted to be there with them, how could all my thoughts be wrapped up in the future state of needing to be back at my desk?

At the start of each day, I would plan how to enter that time with anticipation and gratitude. Thinking, "This is one of the most special times of my day." I would repeat, "I want to be here. I choose to be here." And "I will focus my attention on them during this time." My kids didn't suddenly become effortless to wrangle as we prepared to get out the door, but I started to enjoy and savor the process. I wasn't completing a task. We were sharing an experience. My thoughts were growing in alignment with my values, and it gave me peace.

Execute Your Plan

To get out of "recovery mode" and accomplish a default state of presence, we must continually reinforce the thought that we are right where we want to be. At every interaction, every meeting, and every activity that we engage in, "I want to be here" is our default thought to combat anxiety. It's also our default thought for presence. As we learned in the previous chapter, presence and anxiety are opposites. In fact, anxiety is defined by our *lack* of presence. If we can achieve a fully conscious, fully present day, anxiety has no room to operate. "I want to be here" is the foundational thought to ensure that in big moments and small alike, our performance matches our potential because we have shown up as fully present, devoting our mental resources to delivering in the moment.

Now, it's time to take the concept of our "default thought" to the extreme. Try an experiment where you go through an entire day in everything you do, repeating the thought, "I want to be here." Do it proactively and intentionally at the start of each new activity so that it doesn't end up as a reminder or recovery mechanism when your focus has already slipped. Proclaim those words as a fact. "I want to go for this run." "I want to play with my kids." "I want to eat this meal with my family." "I want to attend this meeting." "I want to work on this report." Don't just do it for the big-ticket items, either. State it before the little things. "I want to get the mail." "I want to open the door for my spouse." "I want to read this e-mail." Then, appreciate that you are where you want to be and doing what you want to be doing.

Before our 2020 move to Southern California, I would go into the office every day, including Fridays, when most of my colleagues worked from home. When we made the move, I abruptly went from five days in the office to none. I had more balance and was protective of the additional time with my family. As work travel patterns returned to normal, I often turned down business trips to stay with them. When I felt compelled to travel, I would go begrudgingly. I joke with Suzy that she thinks of my work trips as "work vacations" because I get to talk with adults and go out to dinner. In trying to convince her that these are hard days, filled with challenging work and tiring hours, I got myself into the mindset that I didn't want to be there. I would attend and do my best to be present, but most of the time, I looked forward to it being over and when I could return to Suzy and our kids. There was nothing wrong with missing my family, but

I was fast-forwarding through days of my life and experiences that could have been meaningful.

As I leaned into the process of shaping the right thoughts, a five-day trip to our headquarters came up for a workshop that I knew I needed to attend. I would not miss the chance to make the most of these days. The agenda called for me to lead a session with a large group, participate in group discussions, and listen to various speakers at different points. The anxiety challenge for me shifted over time from lasting worry connected to formal presentations to momentary stress tied to unplanned communications and off-the-cuff interactions. Tell me I have to present to a few hundred people, and I'll be nervous, but I know I have a process and experience that will allow me to show up prepared and to succeed. Put me on the spot with a random question in front of that same group and queue the fight-or-flight response.

For this trip, I decided my mantra for the entire week would be, "I want to be here." I would show up to each session eagerly as I repeated the thought. I told myself I wanted to be called on. I wanted to participate and to be in the middle of the action. I committed to being proactive. In the past, I may have been more reserved in the group sessions, waiting for my planned time to speak. Yet this time, I was one of the people consistently making observations and asking questions. My thoughts were, "I'm not here to hide. I'm here because I have a valuable perspective to share, to make an impact, and to help us leave here on the path to growth and collective accomplishment." It felt good to lean into the conversation instead of counting the hours to when I could return home.

This trip was an example that transformed not only my anxiety about workplace interactions but the entire experience of the five days. Instead of begrudgingly taking this trip, I was intentional about every interaction, constantly reminding myself I had chosen to be there and wanted to be there. That mindset extended to the hallway conversations, the dinners, and the time in the hotel.

I'm an introvert, so there's often a sense of social anxiety I experience. The source of your energy distinguishes introversion and extroversion. Does a social gathering at work leave you feeling energized or drained? I typically feel drained, even when I have a good time, but I recognized the underlying thoughts in these social settings: "When can I leave?" and "I don't want to be here." Taking the mindset of "I want to be here" through each scenario transformed and lightened my experience. I was still tired after several working sessions or a social gathering, but I also felt a greater sense of fulfillment. When Suzy called to check in, instead of telling her how hard the days were, I told her I was enjoying the time. I didn't rub in the "I want to be here" sentiment, as I empathized with her challenge of managing our three kids alone, but I was done framing my experience in a negative light.

Activate Your Thoughts

While our thoughts form the basis of our behaviors, we can't solely rely on thinking our way to presence. If you're in a half-day meeting just listening the entire time, you'll get bored, your mind will wander, and you'll lose focus. At home, if your family is sitting around the dinner table talking and you're not saying a thing, your thoughts may drift towards the challenging situation you didn't entirely resolve at work that day. Suppose you're meeting with a single other person, and the "conversation" is playing out more like a monologue led by your counterpart. In that case, you'll initiate a conversation with yourself, ignoring the person right before you.

Being in those situations and simply repeating "I want to be here" will fall flat if you don't activate the thought with your actions. If I take my kids to the amusement park, they don't walk around just marveling at the engineering feats represented by the loops and dips of the rollercoasters. They run to get on those rides. Their presence is made manifest through their actions. When they're riding, it's pure presence and joy.

Now, there are two situations where they still might get anxious. The first is waiting in the lines. Just as with adults, their anxious feelings result from their lack of presence. Their internal discomfort is that they want to be on the ride in the future, yet they're stuck in this line. The second potential for anxiety is if they're on the rollercoaster, which is *slowly* making its way up before the first big drop and rush of speed. Once again, the fear, stress, and anxiety are building not because of the slow ascent they're experiencing but because of the anticipation of the rush to come. What's the cure? In the lines, take the action to engage your kids with a conversation or game. During the rollercoaster's slow ascent, focus on the view of the landscape revealed as you climb higher.

In the presidential debate between George Bush and Bill Clinton, both men's actions before speaking foreshadowed the quality of their responses. In Bush's case, his action was subconscious. He turned away from the questioner as he checked his watch, hoping to be done with it all and effectively handicapping his ability to perform to the level that matched his capabilities. For Clinton, his actions were intentional. As the questioner spoke, he sat attentively and faced her. His posture was strong as he held her gaze. Before responding, he made the powerful gesture of standing up, walking into the audience, and engaging her face-to-face. He had no choice but to be present based on his actions.

What behaviors do we exhibit when we want to be somewhere? We engage. We ask questions. We comment on what the other person is saying. If you find your attention beginning to wander in a meeting or other interaction, look for your opportunity to jump into the conversation. It will be impossible for your mind to wander off once you're actively contributing. You don't want to be the person who speaks just to hear yourself talk, but you're in that meeting for a reason. Is it just to sit there and consume or to contribute? When we contribute, our focus is locked in. Why wait for someone else to call on you and put you on the spot? Pre-empt being put on the spot, and you're in the driver's seat.

Even if it's not the appropriate time in a meeting for you to speak up, start thinking about what you *will* say when the time is right. Eagerly await when you can offer a comment or ask a question. Then, when someone calls on you, you're already ready with your contribution instead of being brought into a conversation cold and on someone else's terms. The beauty is that no one else can control what you say when you have the floor. Suppose a question is posed to you that you don't have the answer to. In that case, you can acknowledge it but use the opportunity to redirect the conversation toward the salient point you were eagerly waiting to offer. Participation yields presence and can help us combat anxiety as we flip from a 'be quiet and hide' mentality to a 'lean in and influence' approach.

***

Lack of presence not only opens the door for anxiety to creep in; it also stifles our performance. We can't be at our best when we're not present. Create a schedule optimized for presence. The more significant moments require time for preparation you can carve out in advance. Don't steal your focus from other engagements by worrying about what's ahead. Where you've chosen to be physically, be there mentally as well. Establishing the right environment for presence lays the foundation for your planned thoughts to have their intended effect. You prepared the right thoughts through your morning routine. Now, go and execute that plan.

Take your default thought, "I want to be here," to the extreme, declaring it before every interaction in your day. See how it transforms your experience. Do you find yourself in situations where you're just along for the ride, letting your mind wander as you stare blankly out the window? Wake yourself up and engage to force a state of presence. Participate, ask questions, and pre-empt being put on the spot by engaging yourself first. As your presence grows, the required effect is that anxiety will fade; you leave it no choice as joy and fulfillment take its place.

Chapter Five

Do You Want to be Here?

Where do you have to be today? After my morning run, I have to be home to start my workday, respond to messages, or work on a project before the kids get up. Then, I have to ensure my kids are awake, help them get dressed, and get breakfast. I have to take them to school. I have to get back to my desk and get into the workday. There are meetings I have to attend, messages I have to respond to, and deadlines I have to meet. I have to do all that and a lot more.

Or do I? Do I actually have to do any of that? It turns out I don't. In fact, I am *choosing* to do all of those things. Yet when I establish a narrative of "I have to," I am giving away my power and control. My "I have to" thoughts drive a belief that I am a passenger rather than a driver. That my day and time are dictated by someone or something other than my choices. If my entire day is colored by thoughts that I am forced into various actions, that perception diminishes my experience during those activities. The "I have to" lie primes us for lifeless engagements and outright negative experiences. The truth is that I don't have to do any of it.

Now, I'm not taking this concept to the point of irrationality. If I claim that I don't "have to" take my kids to school, it's true that their lives are not at stake if they miss a day, or two, or ten. However, assuming that we want to provide them with the benefits of an education and school experience, we need to find a way to get them there. But there are options. We could find a carpool to join. We could arrange our schedules so that my wife could take them. They're getting old enough to walk or take a scooter or bike. I take them because I want to take them. I want to have that experience with them in the morning. I chose that the way they get to school is by me driving them. Therefore, it is an incorrect statement that "I have to take them to school."

For your job as well, there was a point before you were hired when you wanted to have that job. You chose to take that position and the duties that came with it. If you now "have to" work a job you don't like, or you find that you begrudgingly "have to" complete all this work that you don't want to do, the reality is there was a point when your mindset changed. That change could have happened on day one of that job, but there was a moment when you shifted from "I choose to" to "I have to."

An essential point to clarify on this book's premise is that I'm not describing a method to remain in a bad situation, but just to feel better about it. If you are in a situation you don't want to be in, change it and opt-out. But own your choices. Own your choices to show up, stay in your job, take on that project, or check your e-mail. "I want to be here" cannot be an empty statement. It needs to be genuine, factual, and a core belief.

"Wanting to be here" doesn't mean that everything we do has to be the equivalent of going to Disneyland *(side note: I use Disneyland as an example that probably brings most people joy, but I really can't stand that place).* We'll explore two critical steps required to optimize how we spend our time and ensure there is truth behind the "I want to be here" mentality. The first is to ruthlessly prioritize and delete any activities that are non-essential, non-value-adding, or genuinely are "that bad." The second step is that when we find ourselves in a sub-optimal situation but it's impractical to opt-out, we need to connect to a larger purpose driving why we are carrying out that activity. In other words, we'll explore when and how to change our behaviors and identify when we should change our thoughts and attitudes instead.

Delete Non-Essentials

Elon Musk has an insane schedule. He works seven days a week, doesn't take "unplugged" vacations, and works from when he wakes up until he goes to sleep. You're probably thinking I could pick a better example if I'm about to talk about work-life balance *(not to mention a less controversial figure, but stick with me).* Yet, you can make a strong case that Musk is one of the most efficient people on the planet. He holds the equivalent of half a dozen or more full-time jobs. At the time of this writing, he is the CEO or de-facto leader of 6 organizations valued in the billions: Tesla, SpaceX, X (formerly Twitter, where he remains the Executive Chairman and Head of Product, despite handing over the CEO role), xAI, Neuralink, and the Boring Company.

Those companies have major subsidiaries that he also leads, such as Starlink in the case of SpaceX and SolarCity or Tesla Solar in the case of Tesla. He also runs a charitable foundation.

Musk doesn't lead these companies in name only. He is intimately familiar with the details of each venture. He considers himself more of an engineer than a business leader, contributing critical design and engineering decisions to each company. As an example of his attention to detail, in his Musk biography, Walter Isaacson described how Elon exercised trial and error to decide how many individual nails were needed to secure each tile on Tesla's solar roofs.[1]

The valuations of Musk's companies alone speak to their respective impacts and accomplishments. Tesla is currently the most valuable car company globally, having disrupted the auto industry with similar aspirations for the broader energy landscape. SpaceX is one of the most valuable private companies in the world and was the first private space company to reach orbit. Not to mention that before these ventures, Musk created a company that disrupted the phone books and influenced other advances in mapping technology and advertising (Zip2), along with another startup that shifted the landscape of the finance industry (X.com, which merged as an equal with PayPal). While Musk could probably use a little more vacation time, you'd be hard-pressed to find someone not just today but throughout history who has had more impact per time spent.

How can one person carry such a load? Part of the answer is what Isaacson refers to as Musk's "algorithm." There are five steps to the algorithm. The first is to question every requirement, even those directly from Musk. Musk found that processes often become bloated with nonessential or nonsensical "requirements" that people don't think to question. The second step is to delete. Once you have exposed the "requirements" that are nonessential, subtract those parts of the process.

Back to the example of the number of nails in the Tesla solar roof tiles, the former SolarCity division was losing money. Musk dove into the roofing process to optimize efficiency and cost. Musk preaches making aggressive cuts when going through the "delete" process. He believes you haven't cut deeply enough unless you find you've gone too far and must restore 10% of what you removed. In the case of the roof tiles, he pushed the team to try securing each tile with a single nail. He relented to allowing *two* nails once he had proof that two were required. His team would not have identified the minimum requirement had they not first gone below the base threshold.

The remaining steps in the algorithm are to simplify and optimize, accelerate cycle time, and automate, but the first two steps are the most essential. For steps three through five, Musk relates how he mistakenly took steps in the Tesla factories to simplify, accelerate, and automate steps or processes that really should have been removed altogether.

The algorithm Musk advocates is upheld in his companies' manufacturing processes, administrative functions, and is even evident in the final products presented to consumers. Take the interior of a Tesla, for example, where a single, large, and sleek touchscreen entirely replaced the myriad physical knobs and dials of most cars. The principle doesn't stop with those functions. Upon his takeover of Twitter, Musk laid off approximately 80% of the company's employees during the initial months of his tenure. While the layoffs were widely criticized for reasons ranging from lack of empathy to the impact on platform stability, Twitter or X didn't fall apart. The service continued to operate (Twitter was probably more infamous for platform instability before Musk's takeover than after), new features were introduced, and most top content contributors remained with the platform. A steep drop in advertising spend was more likely driven by a response to Musk's social and political leanings rather than product degradation. In true Musk fashion, he hired critical employees back in cases where he cut too deep.

While we are almost certainly operating on a different scale than Elon Musk, we can apply his algorithm to our work. Greg McKeown shows us how in his book *Essentialism.*[2] In the book's opening, McKeown paints a compelling picture of a hyper-stressed Silicon Valley executive who is burned out and considering quitting but adopts an essentialist mindset to transform his experience. The executive is advised by his mentor that instead of quitting his stressful job, he should keep working but only do the work he would choose to do as a consultant and opt out of everything else. The mentor also instructs this senior leader to avoid telling anyone about the experiment. The implication is that the executive would complete only the essential tasks while ignoring the rest.

He took the advice and began to evaluate every request by the criteria, "Is this the very most important thing I should be doing with my time and resources right now?" If the answer wasn't "yes," he would turn the request down. This leader began not only turning down non-essential requests but also non-essential meetings, ignoring non-essential e-mails, and no longer signing up for optional projects. He was pleasantly surprised to find no adverse consequences of his new approach. Instead, as he focused only on work that was important to him and of true significance to the company, he achieved better results, received better feedback, and began to regain gratification through his work that, until that point, had slipped away. In this true story, McKeown shares that by focusing only on the essentials and cutting out everything else, you can work less while having a more significant impact.

To apply the essentialist approach, evaluate your upcoming meetings, especially recurring ones. Avoid a sense of pride when assessing, "Do I really need to be there?" If you need to have that meeting, does it need to be weekly? Does it need to be an hour? Could someone else fill in for you? Is a rotation possible among other members of your team? Consider your responsiveness to e-mails and instant messages as well.

I value building a brand of hard work and responsiveness, but establishing that perception does not require a universal approach, particularly to lower-importance communications. Suppose an executive reaches out to me directly. In that case, it's a good idea to get back to them as soon as possible, at least acknowledging that I've seen the e-mail and will work on an answer, even if a resolution is not immediately available. But my inbox is flooded with messages that don't fall into that category. Few people follow e-mail best practices, so you'll regularly receive messages with low relevance.

Scan e-mail subject lines to gauge the message's importance and scan the contents for mentions of your name. Ideally, conduct this scanning in scheduled chunks during the day to avoid the constant context-switching of reading every message as it appears. You'll get through your e-mails in a fraction of the time, and if you miss something, it will come back if it's important enough. With instant messages, there's an expectation for a more immediate reply. But why? Just because someone chooses to send you an instant message does not mean you need to *instantly* read that message or instantly reply.

Focus on how much time you spend working proactively versus reactively. I could literally spend my entire day reacting to e-mails and instant messages. If I did, I'd allow others to dictate how I spend my time instead of focusing on the priorities I've intentionally identified in advance. As Greg McKeown states, "If you don't prioritize your life, someone else will."

By reducing my responsiveness to non-urgent e-mails and instant messages, I've also found that a surprisingly high proportion of those communications resolve themselves. People are resourceful, but sometimes not by choice. Many will reach out before exploring alternatives if they think they've hit a wall. Communications with me are regularly resolved with, "Never mind, I figured it out," or others jump in with solutions when multiple people are copied.

Be bold and experiment with cutting too deep to identify the actual threshold of what's required. Don't be flaky or disappear with no communication, but if you think you can avoid that weekly status meeting without a negative impact on the project, contact the meeting organizer. Let them know that you don't believe you're essential for that week or that you have something else important to work on, so you'll skip this meeting or the series or send your update in a few bullets by e-mail.

Shorten meetings where you are the organizer. A universal principle of meetings is that the discussion will expand to fill the allotted time. When people state at the beginning of a meeting, "This should be brief today," it never is. Let the scheduled time be your boundary. And respect that boundary. People tend to blow past the scheduled end time and continue talking. Let them know that your time is up. It doesn't matter if you have another meeting right after or not. Maybe you need that time to work on a project, prepare for a presentation, or even take a break. Judge for yourself how your time is best allocated.

In the tech industry, working 50, 60, or 70 hours or more per week is standard. The days are typically packed with back-to-back meetings, with nights and weekends being when you can finish your actual work. I have fallen into this trap for years. You find yourself expecting to get nothing done during the day, anticipating that you'll catch up on anything you need to produce in the evening. How can you generate meaningful outputs when you're in meetings all day? Are those meetings really helping the company to grow? To sell more? If those meetings didn't happen, would there be any negative impact on the business? What would happen if I stopped working at night and held a firm boundary that I wouldn't work past 5 p.m.? If I prioritized getting my work done over saying "yes" to everything that found its way to my calendar, inbox, or messaging platform, I would have no choice but to cut out all those non-essentials.

If we want our work to have an impact without sacrificing balance, we need to cut the fat. This process of deletion applies to project prioritization as well. Identify your most important initiatives. Focus on doing a better job on those priority projects rather than spreading yourself thin on many initiatives of mixed importance. As McKeown observes, "Instead of making just a millimeter of progress in a million directions, [you can] generate tremendous momentum towards accomplishing the things that [are] truly vital."

In the book *The 4-Hour Work Week*, author Tim Ferriss describes how his business, selling supplements to boost performance, drove him into the ground.[3] The hours were getting longer, and the results were more difficult to come by. His ambition to own a successful business had become a crushing weight. Tim Ferriss was inspired by the Pareto Principle to break out of his funk, which states that 80% of the outcomes are generated by 20% of the inputs. Ferriss found that very few of his customers generated the lion's share of his business's revenue. On the flip side, most of the complaints that weighed on his time and energy came from a minority of his customers. He had an insight: focus on the 20% of customers that drove his revenue and profitability while ignoring the rest. Sure, he would still sell his product to other customers, but he would do it on his terms. If they pushed, complained, or were otherwise difficult, they were free to buy someone else's products. A surprising thing happened: Ferriss kept most of his customers (including the former difficult ones he no longer catered to), increased his financial success, and drastically cut his hours.

Inspired, he began applying the 80/20 rule to other areas of his life. These included eliminating most of the activities that didn't contribute to his fulfillment, ridding himself of many physical possessions that were no longer necessary, and focusing on learning the 20% of a new skill or discipline that would yield most of the results (including winning a Chinese kick-boxing championship). In addition, Ferriss started a relentless drive to automate or outsource his remaining tasks at work. He eventually reached a point where his previously all-consuming business now occupied such a small amount of his time that he was free to travel the world and generally do whatever he wanted while the company ran itself.

***

In the examples of Elon Musk, Greg McKeown, and Tim Ferriss, all three apply extreme prioritization, the elimination of any non-essentials, and a drive for efficiency in what remains. For Greg McKeown and Tim Ferriss, these essentialist principles open the door for greater balance in life. For Elon Musk, the approach allows him to do the jobs of a dozen people, but hey, if the guy wants to get to Mars, vacations on the beach probably won't get him there.

What is something you've wanted to do but feel you don't have the time? For me, I love living an active lifestyle but working a desk job makes it difficult. As I advanced further in the tech world and the hours crept up from 50 a week to 60 to 70, it felt like I didn't have time to get a haircut once a month, let alone carve out time for fitness *(side note: I cut my hair myself in about 10 minutes and I genuinely struggled to fit this activity in, which gives a sense of the imbalance I had created)*. I remember telling my wife that I felt like a machine programmed to work, strive, and struggle. I had a stretch of over a year when I would work

12 hours a day or more, plus several hours each weekend. After finally finishing my work, I would run outside and work out at a park at around 10 or 11 p.m. in complete darkness. I suspect the coyotes outside our neighborhood considered admitting me to their pack as I passed by each night in the pitch black. I love being active, and it's something I will make fit into my day one way or another, but those night workouts were not a lot of fun.

I didn't change my routine all at once, but I started by scheduling 30 minutes during my workday to work out. Then, I started running to my gym, doing a 10-minute strength workout, and running back. Now I was at 45 minutes. But 45 minutes of activity each day, followed by hours upon hours sitting at my desk, still didn't feel like an active lifestyle. Instead of starting my day with e-mail, I decided to start with my run and morning prayer. Now, I was completing two workouts a day, though I was still sitting a lot. I had always considered sitting on a workout ball instead of an office chair. After years of it being a passing thought, I pushed my office chair to the side one morning and replaced it with the workout ball.

The point is that I just started doing things I previously "wished I could do" or "wished I had time for" that were important to me. I began to prioritize. I pushed physical fitness up my priority list and made the time. I did wake up earlier to complete the morning run and still start the workday early, but the tradeoff was worth it. Applying the essentialist principles at work gave me the space to *make it work.* The knock-on benefit is that exercise during the day cleared my mind and allowed me to work more effectively instead of falling into periods of sluggish energy after hours of staring at a screen. Often, we won't factor in the performance benefits of taking care of ourselves.

There will be tradeoffs when taking control of our schedules. Setting aside an hour in the middle of the day to work out, go to lunch, or see our kid's soccer practice means we won't be available during that time. Success isn't when you get back to your desk and breathe a sigh of relief to see no missed calls or instant messages from your boss. Sometimes, you will return to that missed call from a superior, and, more likely than not, the call came in two minutes after you left. Or, if you decide to go through your e-mails at two scheduled intervals during the day instead of getting sidetracked every few minutes as new messages arrive, that may mean you're not as responsive to every stakeholder as when you're glued to your inbox.

Determine the acceptability of these tradeoffs for your role and identify when your gains in efficiency, focus, and control of your day outweigh the potential downsides. Expect that those downsides will occasionally materialize, but also recognize where the possible drop in perceived responsiveness is more than offset by the enhanced value you will deliver through the quality of your work, ability to execute, and positive attitude you can bring by taking care of yourself.

***

The examples so far have focused on ways to optimize your current situation. Ways to shape an environment through your choices to allow for time and space to focus on what matters. But what if you lack the flexibility or supportive environment that enables you to make these changes? For the most part, if we start saying "no" to lesser priorities, excuse ourselves from non-essential meetings, and prioritize work-life balance, we'll be surprised that our job security doesn't suddenly disappear. But what if you have an overbearing manager who *will* reprimand you for making some of these decisions or even literally fire you? What if you work for a company where the strict policies don't allow for these freedoms? What if the choices enabling you to "want to be there" genuinely are not an option?

We'll cover situations when you can't "opt-out" shortly, but first, have you *tried* to make a change? Too many people accept bad situations when there are alternatives. Is the "I have to" mindset a reality, or is that just what you tell yourself? Have you made it a priority to make a change? What tangible steps have you taken to get yourself in the right environment? Many people underestimate the effort and scope required to make a change for the better. They might say, "Well, I applied for my dream job two weeks ago, and now I'm waiting to hear back." Did you know that 500 others applied for that same position, and no one will even *look* at your application, let alone consider it? Or maybe you're interviewing at a company and want to see how it plays out before pursuing additional options. Did you know ten other people are also interviewing, and it only takes one veto among the 6-person hiring team to take your name off the list? Or maybe in the interview that you thought "went great," the interviewer returned to HR and said, "They did okay. Keep them warm, as they're not my first choice, but maybe we'll reconsider if we can't find anyone better."

You only need one opportunity to work out, but you need to allow probability to work in your favor to land that one. And wouldn't it be better to have two or three offers instead of just one? Apply every day to 40 job postings. Work every major job site in parallel. Research who's doing the hiring. Follow up with the recruiters. Find the hiring managers and send them a thoughtful message. Craft a personal cover letter to stand out, which no one does anymore. Find your connections and your connections of connections that have a tie to that company and leverage them.

I currently work in the marketing department for a large technology company. How many calls and e-mails do you think our cold-calling sellers need to place to reach their goal of setting up six prospect meetings per month? You read that right; I said six *meetings* just to discuss a *potential* opportunity, not actual sales. They need to make 60 calls daily and send 40 e-mails on top of that—every single day. Despite the effort, they won't set up a single meeting on an average day. Doing the math means 1,200 calls and 800 e-mails every month, totaling 2,000 activities. If their goal is six monthly meetings, they have to do over 300 activities to secure a single one. How many attempts have you made again? Are you still waiting for someone to notice that single application? You are on a mission, the fulfillment of which requires a blitzkrieg of activity. Do not accept remaining in a bad situation. Either shape your current situation to meet your needs or find a new opportunity that will.

Find Purpose

Can you honestly say that you've cut out all the non-essentials? What do you now think about those essential activities that remain? If you're honest, maybe some of them still don't seem that appealing. They still look suspiciously like hard work when you'd really prefer to be at the beach or on the golf course. Or you've tried to change your situation, opt-out, or get a different job, but it hasn't happened, at least not yet. Maybe the practicality of supporting your family requires that you stay in a job where the environment is unhealthy. You can't quit that job until you secure a replacement that pays the same. Maybe you can't move on because you're from another country, and your visa is tied to that company. Perhaps you need that specific health insurance. Beyond a job, maybe you're going through a divorce or a serious illness. What do you do *then*? While you keep working or waiting for the right opportunity or your situation to improve, how can you genuinely have an "I want to be here" mindset about a situation no one would want to be in?

Nelson Mandela was one of the leaders of the African National Congress or ANC. The ANC is a South African political party that, in the latter half of the 20th century, focused on bringing equality for black South Africans subjected to racist and segregationist policies known as apartheid. As his involvement in the movement grew and injustice for black South Africans intensified, Mandela was a driving force behind sabotage campaigns aimed at subverting the existing political system and social classes.

Mandela was arrested multiple times, but it wasn't until 1962, several years into his various campaigns, that he was convicted of conspiring to overthrow the government and sentenced to life in prison. Mandela ended up spending 27 years in prison, most of that time at the notorious jail on Robben Island. In his book, *Long Walk to Freedom*, Mandela details the challenging conditions, manual forced labor, and cruel prison officials he encountered over the long years.[4] Twenty years into his sentence, in 1985, as the government continued to confront unrest from black South Africans in the face of injustice, Mandela was offered the chance to be released, provided he denounce violence as a political weapon. Yet, despite the opportunity to gain his physical freedom, Mandela rejected the offer on the basis that he would not enter negotiations while the ANC remained banned and while he was imprisoned.

Did Mandela want to be in prison? No, but he was choosing to be there. He found a higher purpose and mission which, to realize its accomplishment, was worth continued confinement despite the two decades he had already spent behind bars.

Mandela even found ways to experience fulfillment and joy while in custody. In *Long Walk to Freedom*, he shares how the debates with his fellow prisoners strengthened his spirit. He recounts, "These debates were not just intellectual exercises; they were a way of keeping our spirits alive and our minds sharp. We would argue for hours, sometimes late into the night, and these discussions were a source of great enjoyment and camaraderie." Through debate, exercise, pushing back against the treatment of the guards, and even through finding satisfaction in his forced labor, Mandela was able to reflect on his time as having "enriched [his] soul." By way of his mental strength and ability to find joy in the face of difficulty, Mandela emerged from prison without bitterness, resentment, or a thirst for revenge.

After his release, Nelson Mandela went on to be elected president of South Africa in a new democratic and representative process. Upon taking up the position, Mandela focused on bringing unity to *all* South Africans. He worked on behalf of the black and white South African populations, appointing many political rivals or members of opposing factions to leadership positions in his administration.

Nelson Mandela found purpose during his imprisonment, and that purpose transformed his confinement experience, allowing it to play a valuable role in preparing him for the leadership opportunity ahead. Mandela even reached a point where he chose to be in that prison over accepting his freedom. The significance of accomplishing his mission and fulfilling his purpose had surpassed the importance of his release. Most of us will never find ourselves in a situation of that magnitude, equal to 27 years unjustly spent in confinement. So how much more can we connect our struggles to our greater purpose and find meaning and even joy in those hardships?

***

Cognitive dissonance is the distressed state we find ourselves in when our thoughts or beliefs conflict with our actions. We seek to align those two by changing our actions or changing our thoughts and beliefs. The first section of this chapter describes how we can change our environment and actions to alleviate that dissonance. When we can't change our environment, we *can* change our thoughts and beliefs by connecting to a larger purpose.

I've chosen to work a job that requires certain activities that have the potential to give me anxiety, including public speaking. I am good at those activities, though. When I succeed at them, they provide me with fulfillment. They also bring me professional success and financial rewards that allow me to provide for my family. Of course, I'd prefer to do without the anxiety, but I also want the results, the impact, and the success. Claiming you don't want to be present for an uncomfortable activity required to achieve a larger goal is myopic. It may be challenging. It may stretch your abilities. It may feel awkward. However, consider if your short-term discomfort could be outweighed by the potential gains of realizing your larger objective. In that case, the bigger-picture thinking is recognizing that you *want* to engage in that uncomfortable activity.

On the continuum from extroversion to introversion, I am firmly in the introverted category. The Myers-Briggs Type Indicator, or MBTI, is one of the most popular personality tests worldwide, with millions of users. The work of Carl Young, the father of analytical psychology, inspired it. The 2019 MBTI global survey found that the majority of the world's population favor introversion, at 57%. However, the study also found that the characteristics of extroversion are more highly valued for leadership positions, particularly in Western cultures, where 72% of leaders are extroverts.[5] The higher the position, the more likely an extrovert will occupy it.

The findings demonstrate that for introverts to rise in the leadership and executive ranks, many would benefit by adopting some of the behaviors of extroverts, including those that are likely to produce anxiety. For instance, that might mean showing up to a work event that your first inclination is to skip. On the surface, you might not "want" to attend a crowded social event. However, if you aspire to advance in your career, you may recognize that you need a strong network, advocates, and opportunities for influence to accomplish those larger goals. Attending the social gathering allows you to reach the short-term goals that build the foundation for achieving your broader aspirations. If part of your purpose is to grow in your career and you want to do the things that will help you fulfill that purpose, then you can genuinely recognize that you do, in fact, want to be at that gathering.

The Two Types of Purpose

There are two types of purpose, and we need both. There's a "thinking purpose" and a "feeling purpose." The *thinking purpose* is a rational or functional drive. The pieces have a clear and logical connection. We can think of these as "if/then" statements. If we complete the project with high quality and on time, then it brings our team success, helps our business grow, and opens the door for advancement opportunities. If we exceed our work goals, then our potential for personal financial gains increases. If we add a new skill to our arsenal, then it increases our value to the company and broadens our career opportunities.

On the other hand, *feeling purpose* is characterized by a deeper meaning that brings about emotions of passion and excitement. *Feeling purpose* is a motivation that runs through you and gets you out of bed in the morning, eager for what's ahead. If someone observed you conducting an activity driven by *feeling purpose*, they would likely sense your passion. However, it may not be evident *why* you are excited, as the motivation extends beyond surface-level connections. A *feeling purpose* could be an aspirational mission, such as saving lives in the case of healthcare workers. It could be creating a product from which others will derive value. It could be working in the garden of your backyard to grow tomatoes.

While I can provide examples of what both *thinking* and *feeling purpose* may look like, we can all only define for ourselves what constitutes our *thinking* and *feeling* purposes. Neither type of purpose can be put in a box. Some people are driven to climb the corporate ladder, while others are perfectly content with remaining in their current position. Their *thinking purposes* will diverge.

And who can say what drives a person's emotions to create feelings of passion? A project to restore an old car may bring enthusiasm for one person while being considered an arduous task for another. In this way, one person's *thinking purpose* could be another's *feeling purpose*, and vice versa. For example, saying financial gains are only associated with *thinking purposes* isn't necessarily true. What if you grew up in poverty, and the ability to provide over and above for your family fills a deep-seated gap established in your childhood? If you've ever met a good salesperson, you can sense their drive. Their sales pitch isn't one of logic alone; instead, it's based on passion and a belief tied to their offering. These purposes will change over time as well. You may wake up one day and the job you were once excited about has lost its appeal. Your logical reasons for working that job remain, but the fire is gone.

Why do we need to establish both types of purpose? The distinguishing characteristic between the two forms is that they serve different masters. *Thinking purpose* speaks to the logical and reasoning part of the brain, the neocortex. This part of the brain needs a rational explanation for why you're doing what you're doing. *Feeling purpose* connects with our deeper feelings and emotions, residing in the limbic system or what I've referred to as the lizard brain. Both *thinking* and *feeling purpose* need to be established in our work and in how we spend our time to satisfy these two parts of the brain. Absent one motivation or the other, that part of the brain will start pushing back on our actions.

For instance, if you're passionate about under-resourced kids and are working on a project to serve them in your community, you'll be fulfilling your *feeling purpose* and satisfying the demands of the limbic system to connect emotionally to your work. However, what if you work entirely as a volunteer and devote yourself to the project, which makes it hard to provide for your family? Your rational brain will start pushing back, as you are not fulfilling your *thinking purpose*. There may be a middle ground where you find a job that pays a sufficient salary to meet your needs and allows you to serve others in the community. On the other hand, if you work a job because you need the money but can't bring an emotional connection to your profession, your work will feel lifeless as you've been unable to meet the needs of your feeling brain. You'll end up "going through the motions," completing the minimum requirements to stay employed, and watching the clock while you do. You'll still do the work but won't want to be there.

My wife, Suzy, worked in the aviation industry, having gone to pilot's school before transitioning to focus on the business side of aviation. As we were living in Silicon Valley, naturally, Suzy worked at a technology startup that aimed to disrupt the private flight charter business with a new, app-based platform. She was hired to help establish their customer service team. The problem? They didn't have any customers to serve. As the months ticked by, with the product still in various stages of development and the prospect of paying customers appearing like a far-off vision, her role shifted from establishing a customer service practice to managing the office.

As is too often the case in male-dominated industries (and when you combine aviation and technology, that's a double whammy), Suzy became not only responsible for various finance and HR functions but was also charged with establishing a "fun culture," ordering lunches, and keeping the free snacks fully stocked. Their VP of Product practiced a vegan diet, accompanied by a habit of complaining to Suzy that the free food didn't always meet his dietary restrictions. I told Suzy to tell the guy to pay $10 for a salad if he wanted one so badly, but I don't think she ever delivered that recommendation. *(Side note: I eat a mostly vegetable diet myself, which often makes it hard to eat office meals when the default is sandwiches and pizza. But complaining about free food strikes me as a bit entitled and devoid of perspective, particularly when the complaining is directed at my highly skilled wife who has a pilot's license and years of experience leading customer-facing teams and operations functions).*

Suzy was nearly a year into her tenure when we had our first son, Colby, in 2016. She took three months of non-paid maternity leave. We never envisioned being a single-income family and always planned for her to return to work. At the three-month mark, Suzy rejoined her company, and we sent our little guy to daycare. He immediately got sick. And not just a little sick. Being first-time parents, we didn't want to overreact at the first sign of the sniffles, and we knew that exposing Colby to other kids would likely bring about some colds. But after a couple of days of hearing him cough and begin wheezing, we took him to the doctor. He was diagnosed with a respiratory illness called bronchiolitis (kind of like bronchitis, but for babies), where the air passages are inflamed, inhibiting the ability to breathe. The illness required the treatment of a nebulizer, a device where the medicine is administered as a mist inhaled through a mask. It was heartbreaking to watch our baby struggle to breathe. Though the illness is not uncommon, it persisted, returning for spells over the following months.

While Suzy took more time off to care for Colby, she still worked when he was well. By "working," I mean dealing with the complaints of "salad guy." Suzy and I stepped back and thought, "What were we doing?" This wasn't making sense. Yes, Suzy was generating a salary, but her work had no meaning. She had a *thinking purpose* but no *feeling purpose*. And even the *thinking purpose* was growing suspect, as childcare costs consumed a significant portion of her salary.

This period was close to a year after my panic attack. I wasn't an "I want to be here" champion yet, but I was persevering and having success. If I continued to advance in my career, we could comfortably lean into Suzy's higher purpose of raising Colby and, soon to be, two others. *My* purpose became to allow for that to happen. Providing for myself and, subsequently, my family was always a *thinking purpose*. That purpose elevated to a *feeling purpose* when I recognized that my success at work could translate more intrinsically to the well-being of Colby and Suzy. Sure, my salary naturally allowed us to pay the bills, buy food to eat, and pay the rent, but I realized that by succeeding at work, I was buying more than those necessities. My efforts could allow Colby to be in a physically healthy environment, away from the daycare that was the source of his breathing issues, and they could enable Suzy to be in a *mentally* healthy environment, free from the complaints of "salad guy."

What about people's sense of a "calling" in their profession? Doctors might feel called to save lives. Social workers might feel called to help people who are not equipped to help themselves. Scientists might feel called to discover new medical treatments. If you have the "calling" of a particular profession, you have a *feeling purpose*. Alternatively, some companies have a mission that is so compelling it becomes a *feeling purpose* for many of the employees. SpaceX's mission isn't to establish a nice business sending satellites into orbit but to make humanity a multi-planetary species.

Keeping with the space examples, in a 1961 speech to Congress, John F. Kennedy proposed a plan to land a man on the moon and return him safely to Earth before the end of the decade. The following year, in a speech at Rice University, Kennedy made the famous proclamation, "We choose to go to the moon in this decade... not because [it is] easy, but because [it is] hard, because that goal will serve to organize and measure the best of our energies and skills, because that challenge is one that we are willing to accept, one we are unwilling to postpone, and one which we intend to win."[6] The mission united not only NASA but an entire nation, as both the Space Race and the Cold War between the U.S. and Russia were in full effect. There is a famous story, possibly a fable, about a JFK visit to the NASA Space Center in the early 1960s. The story goes that JFK encounters a janitor carrying a broom during the tour. JFK asks the man what he is doing, and the janitor responds, "I'm helping to put a man on the moon."[7] Whether real or not, the story perfectly illustrates the singularity of purpose that an inspirational mission can instill.

You might think, "That's great that I can either have a calling or buy into a company mission, but neither scenario applies to my job." Many workers, and perhaps most, wouldn't classify their profession as a calling, and their company's mission doesn't instill a lasting inspiration. While those two paths to a *feeling purpose* are both powerful, lacking them does not mean *feeling purpose* does not or *cannot* exist. Neither *thinking* nor *feeling purpose* requires any singular source; both types can be multi-threaded and will be stronger if they are.

At different points in my career, I've experienced *feeling purpose* in creating something that didn't exist before, influencing an outcome that helped my company grow, or learning something new that made me stronger. In my profession, I have yet to experience a deep connection to a company mission, nor do I consider my job to be my "calling" in life. I believe my talents are well suited to enable success in my field, but if I had to take up an entirely new profession, I wouldn't feel like I was missing a part of myself by leaving my current job behind.

Would I love to have that sense of calling and deep connection to a mission? Of course, and I am still searching, but it's okay if we graduate college and don't have our life's purpose figured out. I'm 38 years old as I write these words. I am describing how I have lacked a true "calling" in my profession, now more than a decade and a half into my career. Yet, I have struggled, advanced, accomplished, and ultimately experienced fulfillment in my years of work. I have been content with where I am, inspired to reach greater heights, and motivated to do my best work through a combination of *thinking* and *feeling purposes.*

In fact, I am only just discovering the higher purpose in my work through writing this very book. I believe I am sharing an approach that can help alleviate the struggles millions face. I have no idea whether this effort will be successful as I write these words. Maybe this message will reach the masses, or maybe my wife will be the only person to read it. Regardless, I have passion and drive in this work. I will make every effort to make an impact for others who struggle with stress and anxiety, but I will also have peace if it doesn't take hold, as well as confidence that writing this book is a risk worth taking.

***

Malcolm X was a man without a calling through the early years of his adult life. As he describes in his autobiography, he started adulthood as a criminal.[8] Known initially as Malcolm Little, Malcolm X would break into people's homes, steal their valuables while they were away or sleeping, and profit from the sale of stolen goods. After several run-ins with law enforcement, he was caught attempting to retrieve a stolen watch from a pawn shop and sentenced to ten years in prison.

While incarcerated, he experienced an intellectual and spiritual awakening, influenced by other inmates, letters from his siblings, and access to the prison's library. He took the opportunity to educate himself, initially through studying the dictionary to build a foundational understanding of words and their meaning, then gradually expanding to study subjects ranging from history to philosophy to religious texts. Malcolm X also engaged in organized prison debates, deploying his newly expanded vocabulary and honing his public speaking and persuasion skills. After over six years of detainment, Malcolm X was released, having been transformed in his outlook and capabilities. Those years in prison were essential in building the foundation of Malcolm X's influential and inspirational approach, enabling him to become one of the most significant leaders in the Civil Rights Movement.

You may not have realized your purpose, but you may be preparing for it now. It could be that only in hindsight do you recognize that the work you are doing today is preparing you for the future you have ahead. Search for purpose at the two levels: thinking and feeling. Identify where they are established and where they are lacking. But you don't need to feel failure or incompleteness if your *feeling purpose* is not anchored through your life's calling or a connection to a company mission. A major part of life is discovering your purpose. If you haven't found it, don't be disappointed, just don't stop looking.

***

To adopt an "I want to be here" mindset that is genuine, you must pursue both types of purpose *and* become an essentialist. Spending your time efficiently on activities that hold meaning and purpose could be the very definition of where you want to be. If you have narrowed your activities down to the essentials but lack purpose, even the essentials will strike you as unappealing and non-fulfilling. Alternatively, suppose your work has purpose, but you lack an essentialist approach. In that case, you will either become a workaholic devoid of balance, or you will never get to the truly important activities that are most likely to fulfill your purpose. When my two boys were born, I had purpose but lacked essentialism, allowing work to take over too much of my life. This imbalance resulted in missed opportunities to be with them and consumed my attention even when I was with them physically. More recently, I have felt the drive to answer a work "calling" through the writing of this book, but if I allow this project to consume all my waking hours, I'll find myself unemployed and with a family that feels neglected.

As the seasons of our lives change and our circumstances change alongside them, our underlying motivations will also transform. What drove your passions ten years ago no longer gets you out of bed with excitement in the morning. The logical reasoning that has led you to a particular career choice doesn't resonate today. What was an essential preparation activity when you began your career isn't needed anymore, as you have built a base of expertise that you can now rely on. During life's ebbs and flows, regularly reflect on your *thinking purpose* and your *feeling purpose*, and consider the most meaningful activities to participate in each day. We don't need to trick our minds into "wanting to be here." In bringing these three dynamics together, we cultivate an environment where our desire to "be here" is genuine.

Chapter Six

The Higher Call

A surface-level review of this book may conclude its central theme as "the power of positive thinking." That would be an oversimplification. The underlying message is at once harder and more empowering. The ultimate theme is about accountability and ownership. It calls us to recognize that every experience is of our choosing. To accept that if we want to escape the clutches of anxiety, we have to take control of our thoughts. To acknowledge that if we want to show up at our best at work and home, it's our responsibility to be present at each moment.

Do these contentions imply that everything that ails us is ultimately "our fault?" No. There are powerful factors that have shaped you, some of which may include tragedy and trauma. Particularly when considering formative experiences in childhood, you may have had no control over those events, yet they undoubtedly shaped your current mental makeup and life situation. Those things may have "happened to you," but the good news is that by mastering your thoughts, you are in the driver's seat to shape your feelings and actions moving forward.

Adopting this mindset *does* mean we have no one else to blame when our emotions spiral into the negative. How often have you made the statement, "You're giving me anxiety" or "Stop making me angry"? You may not *want* to give up your scapegoats, but taking them away is beneficial. Giving others the power to control your emotions is a life-altering concession. That's your power. Even if many of our feelings derive from the subconscious, we've discovered how to tap into those subconscious processes and alter them by intention and effort.

Yet, while we can take control of our mental and emotional states, we also need the practical realization that complete control of our emotions is borderline impossible. Unless you've reached Zen enlightenment, you won't escape a reality in which other people trigger certain feelings. If your boss chews you out for a mistake or over the perceived quality of your work, you will feel something in response. You may feel offended, angry, or defensive. If your spouse comes home from work in a bad mood and snaps at you, you might feel hurt or compelled to respond in kind. If someone on your team begins panicking about an upcoming deliverable, you're likely to feel a sense of anxiousness growing inside you as well.

Psychologists refer to the transfer of emotional states between people as "emotional contagion." Elaine Hatfield, a professor of psychology at the University of Hawaii, has conducted some of the most widely cited research on the topic. Hatfield notes that psychologists and neuroscientists generally agree that emotional contagion is an innate process (or non-learned) that happens at the subconscious level. This feature explains why it is so challenging to resist adopting the emotional states of others.

Researchers (as well as literally every single parent) have found that infants as young as several weeks will mimic their mother's expressions of emotions, ranging from positive (smiling and happiness) to negative (frowning and anger). That tendency doesn't change over time. What do you automatically do when someone smiles at you? Assuming you're not in a back alleyway at night, you'll likely smile back. If you're feeling sleepy in a conference room and let out a yawn, watch how many others unconsciously do the same. You just infected feelings of sleepiness across the room.

Hatfield found that the process happens in stages, where we first mimic outward expressions, such as postures, facial expressions, and tones of voice. Next is the feedback stage, in which we feel the emotions associated with our mimicry. For instance, returning the smile of another can generate feelings of happiness. Last, we reach the stage of emotional contagion, where we pass on the emotion to others. If someone smiles at us on the street, we're more likely to smile at the next person who passes by. In this way, researchers have found emotional contagion to be more viral than the spread of infectious diseases. Spreading happiness and joy is well and good, but negative emotions can spread just as quickly (and perhaps more easily), including anxiety, fear, and anger.[1]

***

Deepwater Horizon was the offshore drilling rig owned by the drilling company Transocean and leased and operated by the British Petroleum Company, or BP. Nine years into its operation in 2010, Deepwater Horizon drilled an exploratory well off Louisiana's coast in the Gulf of Mexico waters. On April 20th, during the final phases of the exploratory project, a buildup of methane gas shot through the well and burst to the surface, igniting an explosive fire. The fire proved inextinguishable as the flames burned for two days until the rig sank into the Gulf. Eleven workers died, with many others injured, but the devastation was only beginning.

The resulting oil spill raged for 87 days, becoming a national spectacle and environmental catastrophe. Video footage of the oil pumping into the Atlantic Ocean horrified the public. Oil slicks rising to the surface covered over 15,000 square miles at the spill's peak, about 50% larger than the surface of Massachusetts. The spill killed tens of thousands of fish and other wildlife and damaged coral reefs. Residents of the region, spanning multiple states, were exposed to harmful chemicals that were linked to physical illnesses and contributed to mental ailments. Homes were damaged, and property values tumbled. Over a thousand miles of coastline from Texas to Florida was contaminated. An entire region heavily reliant on tourism was economically devastated. All told, over 3 million barrels of oil spilled into the Gulf, which is over a hundred million gallons. The effects are still felt over a decade later, with residents reporting chronic respiratory illnesses (among other ailments), wildlife continuing to be impacted by the remaining oil, and soil with oil contamination levels several times above the average.[2,3]

The offshore rig operator, BP, and their CEO, Tony Hayward, took center stage during the crisis, as oil gushed into the Gulf for months. BP had a poor safety record when Tony Hayward took over as CEO in 2007, having incurred record fines for safety violations in the preceding years. Upon his appointment to the CEO position, Hayward claimed that safety would be their top priority. Three years later, he found himself in the middle of a safety failure of epic proportions.

How did he handle the situation? For any public figure, it's easy to cherry-pick quotes to position them in terms of extremes: as bad or good, capable or inept, or strong or weak. Hayward did say many of the right things during the crisis. For instance, he asserted that BP would be with the people of the Gulf to help them restore their lives long after the reporters had left and moved on to other stories. However, a string of quotes, interviews, and judicial hearings throughout the months-long spill shined light on his true inner thoughts.[4]

Within two weeks of the spill's beginning, the New York Times reported that Hayward confided and complained to his fellow BP executives, "What the hell did we do to deserve this?" Then, he began a series of statements to frame the impact as being blown out of proportion. He stated in early May, "The Gulf of Mexico is a very big ocean. The amount of volume of oil and dispersant we are putting into it is tiny in relation to the total water volume." A week later (and a month into the ongoing spill), he claimed that the impact would prove "very, very modest." At the end of May, the campaign to minimize the event's magnitude continued as he claimed, "The oil is on the surface. There aren't any plumes." Then, in June, as the scope of the crisis became undeniable and public outrage continued to mount, he shifted the blame, stating, "The responsibility for safety on the drilling rig is Transocean. It is their rig, their equipment, their people, their systems, their safety processes."[5]

Two months into the spill, Hayward was brought before a Congressional hearing. During the questioning, committee chairman Henry Waxman asked Hayward whether he felt he had met his commitment to safety, which Hayward claimed was BP's top priority. Hayward immediately responded, "Since I became CEO, we have made a lot of progress." As he tried to continue, Congressman Waxman pushed him to answer the question, opening the door for an admission that BP had failed to live up to their safety ambitions. Admitting as much would hardly have constituted a revelation, given that oil continued to gush into the Gulf uncontrollably as they spoke. Instead, Hayward stated, "We've made major changes," and then talked about how troubled he was by the current events.

The lack of accountability continued throughout the hearing. As questioners confronted Hayward with a long list of concerns about the design of the well and safety compromises made against recommendations, his first response was, "I wasn't involved in any of the decision-making." He placed the blame for the decisions related to faulty design and engineering at the feet of his technical team.[6] After the hearing, whether it was his decision or not, Tony Hayward handed over control of the spill response to executive Bob Dudley.

In what became Hayward's most infamous statement during the crisis, he told a reporter, "There's no one who wants this thing over more than I do, you know. I'd like my life back." That is hardly the most considerate thing to say, given that almost a dozen of the workers on Deepwater Horizon *actually* lost their lives, while thousands of civilians with no ties to the oil industry had their lives upended.

Of course, no one would *choose* to be thrown into a crisis, but leadership is exemplified by how we handle challenging situations. Evidenced by his "I'd like my life back" statement, Hayward didn't want to be there. Not wanting to be there, not wanting to own up to the responsibility, and not wanting to lean in to fix the problem became a contagious mindset that infected the rest of his organization.

His personal statements began to align with the official statements made by BP. Instead of recognizing the issue's magnitude and focusing on its resolution, BP engaged in a PR campaign to minimize perceptions of the disaster. BP stated that only 1,000 barrels of oil went into the Gulf of Mexico daily, later conceding it was 5,000, until it was eventually revealed that the accurate figure was more than 35,000 barrels per day.[7] BP denied the media access to the cleanup sites and limited the information released to the public. These minimizations and the restricted flow of information were genuinely harmful, as they delayed the deployment of more significant resources and bolder solutions that could have stopped the spill sooner. BP's efforts to shift the blame were so overt that President Barack Obama felt compelled to state in a national address, "We will make BP pay for the damage their company has caused."[8]

BP should have prioritized fixing the issue and worried about PR damage control later, but protecting their image and their jobs became the focus of the executive team, followed by the company at large. Outside of communications, BP workers and engineers ignored safety protocols and best practices, leading to the well's failure. These shortfalls, lack of accountability, and predisposition to taking shortcuts were engrained in the culture. Hayward may have inherited a company with a poor safety record, but he had three years to turn that culture around before the Deepwater Horizon explosion. Despite his initial claim to have a "laser focus" on quality, his numerous statements during the crisis revealed his true attitude of indifference, which was infectious. While he was not the one to make the engineering decisions that led to the well's failure, he instilled a culture that allowed those decisions to be made.

***

Now, let's take an opposite example of leadership in the face of catastrophe, evidenced by Winston Churchill. In the latter half of the 1930s, a Hitler-led Germany began a series of breaches of the Treaty of Versailles, which had laid out the peace terms and sanctions against Germany to conclude World War I. Hitler remilitarized Germany, and the Germans began expanding their territory in Europe. The French and British governments exercised appeasement policies to avoid war, allowing Germany to gain momentum. Hitler and Germany grew more daring and eventually invaded Poland, which the British and French had committed to defend. Britain and France declared war on Germany in 1939, but the better part of the first year lacked significant military activity from the British. That changed in 1940 when Germany invaded Denmark and Norway. Britain, along with France and Poland, came to their defense but were defeated and forced to withdraw, with the British losing thousands of lives. Shockingly, France would fall to Germany in those same months.

Neville Chamberlain, the Prime Minister of Great Britain during this period, was forced to step down. Churchill replaced him. With Hitler's army storming through Europe, Great Britain faced a moment of truth. As detailed in Anthony McCarten's book *Darkest Hour*, Churchill faced immense pressure from his political allies and rivals to broker peace with Germany and Hitler. Churchill privately wrestled with the option of accepting peace terms and even conceding offshore territories to avoid losing the mighty nation of Great Britain to the Germans altogether. Pressure mounted as the Germans launched airborne attacks on Great Britain, bombing major cities, including London, which killed tens of thousands of civilians.[9]

Despite the dire circumstances and facing his own doubts, Churchill ultimately demonstrated a resolve so strong in the face of overwhelming odds that he rallied a nation and, over time, a collection of Allied countries in the fight against Hitler and Nazi Germany. He exhibited this determination and conviction with passionate and inspiring speeches delivered in the most harrowing moments of the war. As the Germans were overrunning a once-mighty France, over 300,000 British and Allied troops were evacuated from the French port of Dunkirk, ceding control of France in a shocking defeat. While the evacuation was considered a success, the swift fall of France stunned the world and revealed how perilous the situation was for Great Britain.

Immediately after the Dunkirk evacuation, Churchill delivered the following words in an address to the House of Commons, "The British Empire and the French Republic, linked together in their cause and in their need, will defend to the death their native soil, aiding each other like good comrades to the utmost of their strength. Even though large tracts of Europe and many old and famous States have fallen or may fall into the grip of the Gestapo and all the odious apparatus of Nazi rule, we shall not flag or fail. We shall go on to the end, we shall fight in France, we shall fight on the seas and oceans, we shall fight with growing confidence and growing strength in the air, we shall defend our Island, whatever the cost may be, we shall fight on the beaches, we shall fight on the landing grounds, we shall fight in the fields and in the streets, we shall fight in the hills; we shall never surrender, and even if, which I do not for a moment believe, this Island or a large part of it were subjugated and starving, then our Empire beyond the seas, armed and guarded by the British Fleet, would carry on the struggle, until, in God's good time, the New World, with all its power and might, steps forth to the rescue and the liberation of the old."[10]

Churchill wasn't naïve, nor did he hide the truth. He laid out the distressing situation the British and their allies faced. He conceded the inevitable challenges and setbacks that were still ahead. But what doesn't waver is his resolve. His deep conviction was that if his people committed to the struggle, the victory would ultimately be theirs. As he rallied the Allied forces and implored the United States to enter the fight, he also asserted that the British people would fight on for years and, "if necessary, alone."

Compare Churchill's words with the words of Tony Hayward, as Hayward faced down the Deepwater Horizon calamity when he said, "I'd like my life back." Hayward was loath to lean into the struggle he faced. On the other hand, Churchill promised the public his own "blood, toil, tears, and sweat." Were these just words from Churchill and Hayward? No, they were the outpourings of their inner thoughts and feelings. You can hear and feel Churchill's resolve during his speeches. In his famous "blood, toil, tears, and sweat" speech, he emphasizes the word "*sweat*," conveying that he would personally devote everything to fighting the enemy despite confronting what seemed to be an unstoppable force.[11] Facing overwhelming odds, he was all-in.

The words themselves were meaningful, but the power was in Churchill's resolute delivery, which conveyed his purpose. He willed his thoughts and emotions to achieve contagion, inviting the nation to "go forward together with [their] united strength." The videos of Hayward convey precisely the opposite sentiment. Hayward repeatedly assumes a look and demeanor of aloofness, superiority, and detachment. His words and body language manifested his feelings of not wanting to deal with the crisis. While Churchill was ready to lean into the work, Hayward was anxious to move on when the battle was just beginning.

The sentiments of both men were infectious, with opposite implications for their followers. Churchill inspired a nation, rallying the necessary support of the public, political leadership, and the troops to all fight with passion and tenacity against a powerful foe that overwhelmed every opponent. Hayward's public appearances instilled an institutional lack of accountability, a pattern of blame and defensiveness, and a focus on optics over action. These attributes permeated his organization and allowed a devastating oil spill to continue for months. The feelings both men conveyed in public statements were an outflow of their thoughts. Those thoughts shaped the use of vast resources in both cases. With the oil spill and during World War II, devastation was inevitable, but victory was achieved in only one of those circumstances.

Both Churchill and Hayward started with an opportunity. That opportunity was to put up a fight, to struggle, and to have the chance to persevere in the face of adversity. To take the hard road, but the one that led to a more meaningful outcome. In *Darkest Hour*, author Anthony McCarten recounts how, as Churchill assumed power, he faced moments when he contemplated a compromise with an evil force. He wrestled with those thoughts. The difference between how the two men responded is that Hayward never accepted the challenge. His choice, or non-choice, infected his organization, while Churchill consciously decided to rise to the challenge. Churchill's deep belief in their cause and willingness to do whatever it took to achieve victory defined his time in power and shaped his rhetoric through the war. With the words he chose and the conviction with which he delivered them, there is no doubt that Churchill believed them. He wasn't putting on a show; he was speaking from his soul and choosing to inject a nation with the same steadfast resilience that had become instilled in his mind.

***

In his book, *The 48 Laws of Power*, Robert Greene names "the power of infection" as his tenth law.[12] In alignment with the emotional contagion research, Greene describes how emotions are highly infectious and are transferred from person to person. He advises associating yourself with people who can infect you with positive qualities. If you are lacking in a particular area, they can compensate for that deficiency with their strengths. If you are stingy, for example, associate with those who are generous, and they will unlock your generosity.

He shares how the French nobleman Talleyrand, a seasoned diplomat during Europe's Age of Enlightenment, infected Napoleon's leadership capabilities, significantly contributing to his rise. Napoleon came from a humble upbringing, where his family struggled financially. His early success was based on merit in military campaigns, but to rise as a leader on the national stage required a political intelligence that he did not possess as a younger man. Talleyrand filled that gap, and Napoleon grew in his capacity for adept diplomacy and displays of political acumen through close association with Talleyrand.

While the right connections can serve to build-up our shortcomings, Greene's main message when recounting the "power of infection" is to stay away from people who share your faults, lest they be accentuated; to avoid those who make negativity their default state, lest you drown in misery yourself; and to shun those who practice harmful habits, lest you adopt them as your own vices. Though Greene's message focuses on surrounding ourselves with the right influences and avoiding the wrong ones, what if we flip around the application and look for opportunities to infect others through our positive thinking?

The power of this idea is revealed when we state the relationship more explicitly: we have the opportunity to shape the experiences of others simply through our thoughts. In my home, my thoughts are the starting point to influence a better life for my wife, Suzy, and our kids. This concept may strike you as an overreach. How can we shape another person's experience through the electric impulses running through our brains? The idea may seem on the border of arrogance, but that declaration doesn't need any pride or bravado. If anything, there should instead be an appreciation for the tremendous responsibility it signifies. It's a more profound recognition of the connected chain of activities that leads to the happiness of our loved ones.

If we think the right thoughts, we shape the right feelings for those we care about. Those feelings become contagious in others, and contagion produces the interactions we want. We've all heard the phrase, "I can think my way out of this." We can think our way out of challenging situations, but we can also think our way to a better life for the people who mean the most to us. The opposite implication should be just as motivating. If we allow the *wrong* thoughts to continue, we become a *detriment* to our family's wellbeing. While the connection may be most significant in the context of family relationships, the concept can and should extend to our relationships at work and to addressing the anxiety we face.

The potential for our thoughts to improve the lives of others is appealing, but it also presents a higher call for accountability. Do you perceive a nasty attitude in your significant other? What negative thoughts are *you* harboring towards them that show up in your interactions and return to you as malice? What about the continual disrespect and disregard for your rules that your kids exhibit? Do your underlying thoughts declare that they are good inside or that their character reflects their negative actions? Or take your boss, who doesn't trust you even in the small things and is constantly micromanaging. What negative thoughts do *you* allow to pervade your psyche, which show up in your body language and micro-expressions, coloring your exchanges and damaging your overall rapport?

With Churchill in the case of Great Britain and Hayward in the case of BP, their thoughts inspired the actions of others. Churchill imparted his resolve and belief in the certainty of victory through intention. On the other hand, Hayward was likely unintentional in shaping his thoughts, and his transference of blame and negativity were unconscious implications. Our attitudes will spread to others, whether through intention or negligence.

Consider the essential relationships in your home and at work. That will not be every connection, but focus on those that are (or should be) more lasting: the relationship with your significant other, your kids, your boss, and your teammates. Examine where negativity is embedded. Consider what you believe to be the source of any harmful dynamics. Chances are you ascribe the cause of the negativity to the other person. Flip the script. Identify and take ownership of the negative thoughts *you hold* towards those individuals. You aren't responsible for the other person. Take ownership of yourself and your thoughts and attitudes.

When I was a kid, one of my chores was mowing the lawn. The motor on a lawn mower is loud, and I often used that noise to drown out my grumbling as I completed the task. One day, as I must have been particularly vocal in my complaints, yelling as pebbles flung from the mower blades into my face, my Dad came outside and scolded me. He told me that it didn't matter if I was doing the work if it was done with a bad attitude. I'd love to say that I learned my lesson right then, but the truth is that I've struggled with that concept through the many forms that my work has taken over time, including household chores in my married life. Suzy would refer to it as "angry cleaning," where I'd go about cleaning the whole house but in a bad mood. Although cleaning is a shared responsibility, my underlying thoughts as I worked would focus on what *she* was or was not doing compared to my efforts. Those thoughts would inevitably come out in a negative exchange. Why had I become so focused on comparing what we were both doing?

In marriage, one of the biggest pitfalls is seeking "fairness" in the relationship and, particularly, the fallacy in pursuing a 50-50 split in the division of labor. I've fallen into this trap with Suzy. I would reflect on my duties and compare how they stacked up with her efforts. I ruminated on those conclusions, and the thoughts produced feelings of inequity. The reality is that Suzy is one of the hardest working people I know. But when you enter comparison mode, everyone thinks they're doing more than their share. I didn't want to be in this pointless cycle. I started to think back to when we were first dating. Back then, I took pleasure in everything I did for her. I wanted to lighten her load. To serve her. To do things for her to make her life easier. You could argue that I *did* far more of those things now than when we were dating, but my attitude had significantly shifted.

I also recognized that while I tended to complain, I had the strength and capacity to take on even more than what I was doing. I didn't need to "decompress" after work. I could jump right in with the kids. Doing the housework felt more fulfilling than sitting down and watching TV. My genuine desire was to support Suzy with whatever was needed. In rationally assessing my capacity and willingness to do the work, in contrast with my negative attitude, I concluded that comparing our workloads was pointless. It didn't matter what *she* did. It mattered what *I* did. I began to repeat that I was thankful for having the strength to do the work. I would plan in the mornings to actively seek out opportunities to do things that would be helpful to Suzy during the day. If she asked me to take care of something, that request would signal that I had the chance to do what I genuinely *wanted* to do.

When I do the work begrudgingly or focus on what someone else is or isn't doing, it sours my mood and infects the temperament of our entire house. If I instead focus on myself and choose to take satisfaction in the work, I accomplish even more than staving off my own negative feelings. In replacing the destructive thoughts with a focus on supporting my wife, I not only rediscover the fulfillment that comes from serving my partner; I also generate feelings of joy, purpose, and accomplishment that are palpable to my family and can elevate our shared experience.

Optimizing for harmony with Suzy is one matter; dealing with the three small ticking time bombs of emotion who also live in our house takes the challenge up another level. When my kids start up the roller coaster that is their emotions, it's hard not to go along for the ride. One of our kids tends to go to extremes in negativity if an argument or fight breaks out. "I hate my brother," "I wish he were never born," and "I'm going to throw him in the trash can" are all statements that have been screamed more than once in our home.

Regulating emotions is difficult for adults but even more challenging for kids. The swings from highs to extreme lows can be sudden and dizzying. The herculean challenge is not letting those emotional swings infect us as parents. When my boys start tearing at each other, and the rage pulses through their little bodies, I often feel the grip on my own emotions loosening as I'm sucked into the conflict. These situations are where the responsibility is so great. Given that one of our children is predisposed to go to darker places, my response will either fan the flames or defuse the situation (albeit gradually). It is a terrible outcome if my child runs to their room feeling emotionally out of control when I have contributed to that sense of spiraling. But emotions flare up in an instant, and attempts to "control" them are unreliable. To combat emotional contagion, the effective approach is to focus on the thoughts that lead to that reaction.

Dr. Becky Kennedy is the author of the book *Good Inside*. [13] The fundamental premise is that we must believe that our children are genuinely good inside and outwardly convey that belief through our interactions, especially during challenging moments. Instead of focusing on modifying their behavior, we recognize their goodness, validate their big feelings, and help them navigate through their emotional struggle. In dealing with my kids' emotional outbursts and negativity spirals, I had to examine the underlying thoughts *I* was having in those moments. While the love for my kids runs to my core, in the heat of the moment, my thoughts zero in on the negativity of the behavior exhibited. I think that they are being mean, disrespectful, unreasonable, or some other negative trait (word of advice: never expect young kids to act with reason). Sure, they exhibited undesirable actions, but I needed to shift *my* thinking to focus on my more fundamental and lasting beliefs about them rather than on momentary behavior.

Even amidst an emotional outbreak, I could remind myself that I had good kids who were just having difficult moments. Broadening my thinking was the key ingredient, preparing me to react with poise amid a storm of emotions. As an additional step, I consciously needed to lower my expectations regarding their emotional regulation. Their capacity for reason and logic is years away from fully developing. At times, I recognized that I was levying the expectations of emotional control that are only appropriate for adults, placing that burden onto children who had yet to develop that capacity.

The process of unpacking the unhelpful existing thoughts and purposely replacing them with the right ones should be an intentional and thorough exercise conducted before the next emotional eruption and repeatedly reinforced to ensure it sticks. Successfully priming this thinking pattern can be the difference between an outburst being a brief detour or it ruining an entire day, as one of my kids drowns in big emotions like anger, anxiety, and frustration. Some things won't change. We will still have the emotional outbursts and fights to disrupt, as one of my kids will inevitably "steal" the other's dinosaur, say something mean, or even just look at one of the others for too long. I will still need to step in and manage the conflict. Their emotions will still be dysregulated. But, I can lead with composure and leverage its contagious effects, allowing it to take hold as their emotions peak. Once they're safely separated, I can assure them they are good kids, having a rough moment. I can tell them I love them, even when I don't love their behavior. I can remind them that big emotions can *feel* like they will never go away, but they will pass. As they experience my genuine love, poise, and peace, they will [gradually] begin to feel the same.

At work, we can take the same attitude of extreme owners hip.[14] I've been fortunate with the bosses I've had throughout my career. Even with the good ones though, these relationships ebb and flow. There are always occasions of struggle or conflict. Your rapport with your direct manager is one of the primary drivers of your experience at work. If you are struggling in that relationship, there is a natural tendency to focus on the other person's actions as the source of that frustration.

I found myself in a situation where I felt shackled and micromanaged by my boss. Why didn't they let me run my part of the business the way I saw fit? Why were the projects I believed could move the business forward being disregarded? Why had my opportunities for career advancement suddenly been closed off? I struggled with these thoughts, and they soured my attitude towards work. The problem was that I didn't want to change jobs. I still wanted to be there. So, *I* had to make a change.

I couldn't change my environment, so I focused on changing the thoughts shaping my attitude. I considered the wrong thinking in me. I realized I saw my boss as a rival, not someone I could serve and support, but as someone to compete against. My ego had gotten in the way. I was letting those wrong thoughts color my beliefs about my boss's character. To change the dynamic, I took a page from Dr. Becky's "*Good Inside*" philosophy and began to seed thoughts that my boss was fundamentally a good person. They faced challenges beyond my own and those I knew nothing about. I chose to believe they *did* want to help me and the team but that *I* needed to support them better first.

As I worked to engrain these thoughts, a funny thing happened. My boss seemed to lighten up. The underlying tension in our interactions began to dissipate. As I reframed my view that we were sitting on opposite sides of the table to one where we were sitting side-by-side, I felt more supported in our interactions. It began to be not so hard to believe those thoughts as their truth played out. Where previously I felt surrounded by walls, I now perceived open doors. Had my thoughts and the perception of our relationship changed? Yes, my subjective assessment of the situation had shifted, but so had many of the objective characteristics of our dynamics. Changing my thoughts was the cause that led to the effect of the transformed relationship. The fundamental change wasn't in my boss; the change was in me, beginning with a recognition that *I* was responsible for the situation that I was in and, more encouragingly, that I had the power to change it.

***

Every day, you're likely to encounter situations where the energy in the room is negatively charged, either at work or home. Instead of seeing these as situations to avoid, reframe those settings as opportunities for you to exert your influence. Be like Churchill and throw yourself into the fight. In the case of Churchill, the strength and resolve of one man had the power to shift the attitude of an entire nation from fear to determination.

When we encounter chaos in our homes or at work, we can turn our backs and avoid these challenging situations. Or, we can get swept up in their emotional contagion, going along for the ride. Alternatively, we can rise to the challenge and turn the tide ourselves. Is a team at work feeling overwhelmed by the pressures of a deadline? Step in with poise and leadership, happily grabbing an oar to paddle alongside them, infecting an atmosphere of excitement for the potential impact. Is there a cloud of negativity in your home, stealing your family's joy? Consider it *your* job to step in and light the way. That may mean leaning into their pain or discomfort as a start, but concentrate on how your energy can be the life ring that keeps their heads above the waves and gets them back into the boat. Focusing on the opportunity to achieve a higher purpose can be the fuel that maintains your positive thinking in the middle of a storm.

Chapter Seven

The Train Has Left the Station

We're going to have good days, and we're going to have bad days. As I leave each morning for my run and begin reflecting on any missteps from the day before, sometimes I recognize that I successfully executed my plan, and my focus turns to continuing those right thoughts today. Other times, I acknowledge how I blew it big time and let the wrong thinking overrun me, leading to actions I'm not proud of. Even as we grow in the discipline to shape the right thinking, we'll still have those bad days. And, as our strength builds, we'll raise the bar for what defines our desired thoughts and behaviors, so there will always be opportunities to get better and mistakes to correct. Given that the bad days and patterns of negative thinking are inevitable, what do we do when the train has left the station, and we're spiraling into a sea of negative thoughts?

A flywheel is a mechanism that regulates energy transmission from an engine. That engine can be mechanical in the case of a car, but the engine could also be human in the case of an antique sewing machine. If you've seen movies set in the 1800s, you may have watched scenes of people pumping their feet as they operate these old devices. What they're doing through the foot pumping is propelling a flywheel forward, which feeds consistent energy to the sewing mechanism. A flywheel is challenging to get going, as it is typically a heavy piece of equipment. However, once you get the wheel moving from a concerted effort, momentum takes over, and only small applications of force are required to sustain its operation. Each push from the worker's foot builds on the previous pumps, with the collective energy driving the wheel forward.

An anxiety spiral operates like a flywheel in our minds. We have an anxious thought as an unexpected bill comes in. Next, there are four Amazon packages at the door. Then, we find out that our kid made the traveling team, but it will cost five times as much as their old team. Suddenly, we're in a state of financial distress and all it takes is for our spouse to buy the more expensive name-brand cereal for us to feel overwhelmed. The more expensive cereal purchase was only a minor push, but it built on all the momentum from the preceding events. Anxiety spirals go hand-in-hand with the psychological concept of rumination, in which we continually review and rehash problems in our minds, including the factors that led to those problems and their resulting consequences.[1] We don't reach a conclusion; instead, we keep revisiting those problems, turning them over and over in our minds from different angles.

Going even further than a flywheel, our negative thoughts can reach a point where they are an entirely self-reinforcing system. The genuine inputs that established the momentum (the bill, the expensive traveling team, the grocery purchase) shift to "what if" inputs that we generate in our minds. "What if *another* unexpected cost comes in?" "What if I don't get the bonus I was promised?" "What if I lose my job altogether?" We've entered a cycle that only requires our thinking to accelerate. Momentum has overtaken us, and the force feels too great to stop.

***

While momentum can be positive, its implications can feel even more significant when it is a store of negative energy building in our flywheel. Momentum is often a powerful negative driver in sports, as was the case of Martina Hingis's match against Steffi Graf in the 1999 French Open final. Martina Hingis came into the final as the top-ranked woman in the world and was heavily favored to win. She was only 18 years old at that point but had already won five Grand Slam singles titles. Steffi Graf, on the other hand, was a legend in the sport, boasting a record 21 Grand Slam singles titles. However, she was considered to be in the twilight of her career, having not won a major singles title in three years as she battled injuries (indeed, Graf would go on to retire later that year). Graf came into the tournament ranked outside the top five and even admitted before the match that she was surprised to have made the final.[2]

Hingis took a commanding lead, winning the first set 6-4 and taking a 2-0 lead in the second set. In women's major tournaments, the first to win two sets wins the match, so the victory was in sight. *(Note that 6 "games" wins a set and 2 sets wins a match.*

The hierarchy is game, set, match, from lowest to highest). Hingis was in control and cruising to a championship victory, but then there was a controversial call. With Graf serving down 2 games to 0 in the set, Hingis floated a forehand return to the baseline. The ball is initially called out by the Line Umpire, though the replay shows that the shot appears to have landed comfortably in play. The Line Umpire and Chair Umpire come onto the court to discuss the call. The French Open is played on a clay surface, with the benefit being that the umpires can walk over and look at the marks left by balls striking the clay court, to visibly confirm whether a shot is in or out. After the conference, the umpires upheld the call as "out."

Hingis looks shocked, arguing with the head umpire and crossing to the other side of the court to point at the mark where the ball landed. She refuses to continue play, demanding that a separate tournament referee make a ruling. Hingis can be heard arguing that the umpires were looking at the wrong mark on the court (which they likely were). Her act of crossing the net to her opponent's side of the court is a code violation, and it resulted in a one-point penalty in that game, which she lost. Though still up 2 games to 1 in the set, the momentum, which was strongly in her favor, shifted. The crowd, already leaning in favor of Graf, turned hostile to Hingis. While Hingis maintained a lead in that set and was serving to win the match up 5 games to 4, Graf broke Hingis's serve, winning that game and the next two to take the second set, 7 games to 5. In the third and decisive set, Hingis unraveled, losing 6-2, giving Graf the final Grand Slam victory of her illustrious career.

Although the match was close leading up to the controversial call, Martina Hingis was in control. She was the stronger player at that point in their careers and on that day. But Hingis couldn't move on past the call. She couldn't put it behind her and focus on the next point or the next game, even as she maintained the advantage. It hurt as well that she was facing such a decorated opponent.

Momentum in sports is most apparent when both sides experience it in opposing directions; self-belief in one side surges as their play elevates, while their opponent's conviction dissipates as the mistakes mount. Martina Hingis knew she faced an opponent capable of overcoming any deficit in Steffi Graf. Graf knew what she was capable of as well. In a dialogue that proved prophetic, right as the controversial point was playing out, one of the announcers commented, "Steffi's got to be real careful here this doesn't go quickly in the second [set]. She's going to have to dig deep in the well right now." The announcer's counterpart responded, "You could look at it the other way too... Steffi definitely is match tough... and Hingis was playing a little bit loosely in that first set." The second announcer called it right. Steffi Graf *was* mentally tough and ready for the opening, while Martina Hingis was cracking. The opposing forces of momentum resulted in Hingis's defeat and her unraveling in the third set on a day she had started as the clearly superior player. After the match, Hingis stormed off the court before being brought back for the award ceremony by her mother (who was also her coach) in tears.

The spiral didn't end there. Two weeks later, Martina Hingis, the world's best women's tennis player who had already won five major titles, including one that year, was dominated in the first round of the Wimbledon major tournament, losing 6-2, 6-0 to a 16-year old Australian, Jelena Dokic. Hingis not only lost that year's French Open, but she would *never* win a French Open. In fact, Hingis would never win *any* other Grand Slam singles title after her crushing defeat. Four years later, persistent ankle injuries forced her early retirement. She staged a comeback in 2006 but was forced out again after testing positive for cocaine.[3] She never returned to the form she had enjoyed right up to that moment in the second set of the 1999 French Open final.

The turning point in that final was not physical. Hingis hadn't sustained an injury during play, a common factor in turning the tide of a tennis match. A switch had flipped in her brain. In an interview about a year later, Hingis reflected on the moment, "I think I lost my mind. There was so much pressure."[4] Curiously, the single point that reversed the momentum wasn't meaningful. It was the first point of the game in which Graf was serving. Already up 2-0 and with Graf expected to win her service game, that single game was not pivotal for Hingis, let alone the first point. In addition, Hingis's contested shot hadn't even been a clear winner, so overturning the call wouldn't have given Hingis the point; they would have to replay it at best.

Bad calls happen in tennis, even in the biggest moments. Professionals know that the potential for human error comes with the territory. In most cases, Hingis would have shaken off the bad call. Yet, in this case, Martina Hingis felt the pressure of facing the most decorated woman in tennis history while simultaneously being positioned as Steffi Graf's successor. And Hingis was still only a teenager. The pressure cooker building inside her turned a momentary setback into a career and life-altering moment. Hingis was not only unable to stop the negative momentum in that match, but her inability to turn the page had implications she would feel for years.

Momentum is an intangible force. You can feel and recognize its consequences in sports and life, but it cannot be quantified or visibly observed. Sports psychologists Jim Taylor and Andrew Demick created what they refer to as a multidimensional model of momentum in sports.[5] The model identifies a chain of events leading to shifts in behavior and performance. The stages are: 1) a precipitating event that serves as the trigger or catalyst; 2) a change in thoughts, emotions, or physical state experienced by the athlete(s); 3) a resultant change in behavior; 4) an associated increase or decrease in performance; 5) an opposite change experienced by the opponent; and 6) the end-product, which is a shift in the outcome. These stages parallel the CBT (cognitive behavioral therapy) paradigm, as the trigger sets in motion a chain of events in which new thoughts lead to behavior changes that alter the performance and outcomes in a game. Our thoughts and beliefs ultimately create momentum, and when we believe we have momentum (positive or negative), its effects are real.

Whether it's sports, work, or home life, momentum is a construct created in our minds with real-world implications. Negative momentum plays out during spiraling and rumination. At work, when we're delivering a presentation and start strong, we know we're in control and a positive outcome is assured, even if we're only 10% into the session. However, it can be hard to recover if we stumble at the outset. You might come home after a rough day at work, and it feels like the bad breaks have followed you there or have even accelerated. Maybe you forgot to pick up a kid from practice, got overcharged at the store, and the microwave stopped working. The stress intensifies with each small setback. When the momentum of anxiety is building, we may feel like we're losing control and that a once-certain victory is now slipping away. How do we stop that momentum when it feels like the train of our thoughts has left the station and our conductor was left behind on the platform? No one is at the controls, and we're speeding towards a crash.

Call a Timeout

Calling a timeout is one of the most popular ways in sports to stop negative momentum. The twentieth century brought about the adoption of the modern timeout in professional team sports. However, timeouts have existed for centuries and are even present in sports without a formal timeout provision. In soccer, for instance, halftime serves as a timeout, providing time for rest and adjustments to strategy and tactics. Even during the run of play, and to the ire of fans in the United States, professional soccer players will commonly exaggerate an injury to disrupt the flow of the game and allow for a strategic stoppage. Research has shown that timeouts are effective, as various statistical studies of basketball games indicate that teams subjected to "scoring runs" by the opposing team tend to improve their scoring differential immediately following a timeout.[6, 7]

A notable anecdotal example of the power of a timeout is the 2013 Super Bowl between the Baltimore Ravens and San

Francisco 49ers, which leveraged a very non-traditional timeout. The Ravens built a commanding 28 to 6 lead, which they carried in the second half, presenting what seemed to be an insurmountable advantage. Everything was going right for the Ravens, while the opposite could be said of the 49ers, who had only managed two field goals with most of the game behind them. Then, the lights literally went out in the New Orleans stadium, as a power outage left the players and crowd in darkness for over a half-hour during the biggest game of the year. When power was restored, the momentum abruptly flipped, and the 49ers, who had been inept on offense to that point, scored 17 unanswered points and were a failed 2-point conversion away from tying the game. While the Ravens narrowly held on to win by a score of 34 to 31, the comeback was nonetheless one of the most improbable swings in momentum in Super Bowl history.

The shift in performance resulted from the opposing ways each side perceived the same event. After the game, several Ravens players indicated they believed the power outage was a conspiracy to bring the 49ers back into contention (and they were not joking). On the other hand, several of the 49er players and coaches described the outage as delivering an opportunity to regroup mentally while also allowing for the planning of tactical adjustments.[8] The power outage disrupted the focus of the Ravens while resetting the focus of the 49ers.

A timeout can be the perfect tactic when momentum builds as an opposing force against us. We've all been in situations that feel overwhelming at work. Your boss lists five things you need to do in rapid succession, and they're all "high priority." Perhaps more challenging is when you're in back-to-back meetings and take away urgent action items from each one. The rest of your day is filled with yet more meetings, leaving you with no time to work on the tasks you've already accumulated. Your upcoming meetings will also likely add even more to your overflowing to-do list. You feel like you're carrying a load right on the edge of your capabilities, yet each passerby throws another bag on your back. You can take just one more, right?

We need to focus on the most important activities to have a meaningful impact, but what if we have so much thrown at us that we struggle to identify what *is* most important? When you're overwhelmed, you can't think and prioritize clearly. You might start inefficiently trying to work on three different tasks at once, potentially even ignoring the most meaningful one that sits unattended on your to-do list. Call a timeout to list out everything being asked of you and identify the most critical [*singular*] priority. It may help to include your boss in this evaluation, who will serve the role of a coach. Put the onus of prioritization on them, letting your boss know you have five activities on your plate and the capacity to complete one today. Which one should you choose? Prioritization is one of the most important jobs of a manager, so let them do their job to prioritize your work so you can focus on being effective on the most meaningful tasks.

Recognize that timeouts serve different purposes as well. These purposes include resting, refueling, reviewing a necessary change in strategy, or planning your next move or play. Take the time for what you need. Is your heart racing, and do you need time just to be still? Use the timeout for a few quiet moments of rest. Are your efforts proving ineffective, and are you uncertain how to change the dynamic? Use the time to consider adjustments to your approach. Are you overwhelmed with the enormity of tasks you've accumulated? Use the time to list all your requests, assessing their importance and level of effort to complete. Set a boundary of how much time you can spend working on them. Then, choose what you will work on within your established time box.

One of the most essential purposes of the timeout is to break the momentum of negative thoughts and feelings you're experiencing. Teams call timeouts in sports when their opponents go on a scoring run. With the game paused, the run cannot continue. What is *your* space that can serve to break the momentum generated against you? It may be to go for a run or walk, to play an instrument or listen to music, or to call a friend or family member.

CBT focuses on your thoughts as the first domino, which cascades to your feelings and actions. However, this relationship can be reversed. When our thoughts and feelings are beginning to spiral out of control, a change in our behavior can force a change in our mental state. In our home, my wife and I often find our mental stores have been depleted, and we no longer have the strength to stand against the will of a three-year-old. When we can feel ourselves heading to a breaking point, it's time for a timeout, relying on our partner to take over, or acknowledging the kids will be fine fending for themselves for a few minutes. My wife's preferred timeout is a shower. If I'm completing their bedtime routine and sense that I'm about to lose it, I'll step away to take care of myself for a moment, washing my face, taking my contact lenses out, or doing something else to steal away a few minutes. I use that time to acknowledge my unhelpful, untrue thoughts that emerged as the kids' bedtime revolt played out and replace them with more helpful ones. Then, I get back into the game.

Try to incorporate exercise into your breaks whenever possible. Don't have time to run or even take a walk? Do some jumping jacks or push-ups right where you are for a minute or two. Attempt to engage in aerobic or cardiovascular exercise, which requires increased oxygen intake and an accelerated heart rate. You might think, "Wait a minute, I'm taking this timeout because my heart *has* been racing. When I want to slow it down, why would I intentionally speed it up?" While stress and exercise both lead to a similar outcome of an elevated heart rate, there are different processes and hormones in play, some healthy and others not.

When we're stressed, our fight-or-flight response triggers the release of stress hormones like adrenaline and cortisol, which cause your heart to beat faster, your blood pressure to rise, and your muscles to tense. Remember the problem: our body makes these changes to prepare us to fight or run, yet it's a false alarm. These stress hormones are deployed in excess of the true physical demand. When exercising, we still release stress hormones, but they are balanced to match our genuine physical needs. Exercise also triggers the release of endorphins; hormones that make us feel good. Endorphins block perceptions of pain, relieve stress naturally, and trigger positive feelings. Yes, your heart rate will increase along with your breathing. The difference is that these responses now fulfill a necessary function to deliver the higher blood flow and oxygen required to support your activity level. It's by these processes that exercise serves to clear the mental fog brought on by our stress and anxiety, delivering clarity of thought.

The "answer" to what had just minutes ago seemed to be an intractable problem will quite possibly come to you during a run or brisk walk outside. Let your mind wander as you take each step. Your unconscious will keep sorting through the problem while you let your attention draw towards the scenery you pass by and the bends in the road. As you experience the benefits of the endorphins released in your system and an increased oxygen intake, the solution may suddenly jump to the forefront of your mind without you even trying.

Focus on Breathing

I'm amazed by the range of fundamental and unconscious activities that I'm not naturally good at. For example, I run just about every day of the year, rain or shine. You'd think I would be pretty adept at tying my shoes by now, right? I used to pull my running shoes on, lace them tight, and head out. That approach was sufficient for relatively shorter runs, but there were a few years when I would run a half-marathon distance, about 13 miles, once a week. Once you get to 10 miles and beyond, the little things start to matter. I would have pain in the tendons around my ankles, blisters would form on my heels, and the tops of my feet would ache in pain. One of the main culprits was that I didn't know how to tie my shoes properly. The pressure of the laces was unequally distributed, causing unnecessary strain and aching in my feet and ankles. I laced them too tight at the top, impacting proper blood flow. I wasn't considering that your feet swell during longer runs and need space to expand into. And then I discovered there were fancier ways to tie your shoes, such as creating lace locks to ensure your heel doesn't slip with each step, prohibiting the friction that causes blisters.

I had moved on from thinking about tying my shoes since kindergarten, yet here I was, returning to the fundamentals. It turned out I needed not just a re-education, but there were nuances I had never learned. I continue to discover many more fundamental activities I've been performing sub-optimally. These include how I position my weight when standing, my posture when sitting, my form when running, and more. It's the same with the even more fundamental exercise of breathing.

Evidently, you've figured out how to breathe, or you wouldn't be reading these words now, but that's precisely the point. Many people have established breathing patterns that allow them to sustain their existence but not to optimize their health and well-being. In his book *Breath*, James Nestor outlines many suboptimal breathing practices people have adopted, the impact on their health, and the preferred alternative.[9] He details the importance of breathing through the nose instead of the mouth, as the nose acts as a powerful filtering mechanism and humidifier that the mouth cannot match. In addition, the air that reaches our lungs through our noses delivers about 20% more oxygen than the equivalent breaths inhaled through our mouths.

During a rush of anxiety, we should fight our impulse to take in deep gulps of air through the mouth. That practice introduces more air than we need, overwhelming our system when our real goal is to calm things down. The opposite approach is often the most effective. Taking slow, deliberate breaths through our nose and holding our breath, both once we've filled our lungs and once we've wholly exhaled, can slow our heartbeat and restore the clarity of our thinking. In this way, the opposite act of holding our breath when we feel the need to hyperventilate can be a more effective tactic.

We also need to adopt the correct posture to breathe properly. In yoga or meditation, a significant focus is on proper breathing and positioning our bodies for optimal oxygen intake. When you see someone sitting in a meditative pose, is it ever associated with slouching? No, their posture is erect, and their balance is centered, allowing their lungs to inflate and deflate to their maximum potential. And what is the cadence of their breathing? It is slow and controlled. Anxiety speeds everything up as we go into fight-or-flight mode. Consciously slowing our breathing down, with controlled and full breaths through our nose, not only delivers a more efficient intake of oxygen that our rational brain can leverage, but the deliberate and slow process also signals to the lizard brain that we are okay; there is no danger.

Breathing exercises have two primary benefits. The first is they can relax us when we enter a state of stress or anxiety. Second, they will build competencies in breathing control, train our bodies to use oxygen more efficiently, and enhance carbon dioxide tolerance (the waste product we breathe out). These are capabilities that will help proactively avoid the harmful physical implications of anxiety. There are many different breathing exercises. Try different options. I practice box breathing, where you breathe in through your nose for a slow count of five until your lungs are full. Hold your breath for five seconds, then slowly exhale for the same count until your lungs are empty.

Hold here again for another five seconds before repeating the cycle. Extending your exhale time beyond your inhale time can help you further relax and gain greater control of your breathing patterns.

Exercises like these jumpstart the parasympathetic nervous system, which is responsible for the body's 'rest and digest' responses. The parasympathetic nervous system is engaged during sleep, as our bodies slow our breathing and decrease our heart rate. By taking the active step to slow and control our breathing, we activate that system to leverage its relaxation benefits. The great thing about breathing exercises is that we can practice many of them in front of other people, and they will have no idea we're doing them. Are you about to be introduced to give a talk, and you feel anxiousness rising within you? Establish a strong and balanced posture and execute one of these breathing exercises until it's your turn to speak.

The effective delivery of oxygen affects every major system in the body that we rely on for essential functions and for achieving peak performance. Our oxygen intake directly impacts our heartbeat, our breathing facilitates our blood circulation, and our brain depends on the oxygen delivered by breathing. In the midst of anxiety, we might try to control our thoughts, but negativity can overwhelm us. In that case, go one step further back. Our brain generates our thoughts, but our oxygen intake sustains our brain. The fundamental construct of CBT could be extended as follows: your breath feeds your brain, your brain drives your thoughts, your thoughts drive your feelings, and your feelings drive your actions. Do you want to control your feelings? Start with intention in your breathing.

Do Nothing... Or Actually Just Try Something

What if you can't call a timeout and know you can't breathe your way out of it? Do we have other tips and tricks to employ? Yes, though it's not a trick; in fact, it's nothing at all, literally. When the train is speeding down the track, and you know you can do nothing to stop it, let it run its course. Do you have the impulse to run as an anxiety spiral intensifies? Take the opposite action and stay. But instead of wishing you weren't there, be present in that moment.

The ocean presents a great teacher for dealing with anxiety, both as a metaphor and a method for handling it. Anxiety can wash over us like a wave. The power of the ocean is remarkable, and it's pointless to fight against it. What should you do when caught up in a strong current? Nothing. Struggle gets you deeper into trouble, depleting your strength. What does a surfer do when they fall off their board and get caught beneath a wave? If they struggle against it, they'll use up their breath and may not have the capacity to reach the surface. Instead, if they remain patient, the strength of the current will pass, and they can safely float to the top. In the same way, if you are swimming in the ocean and find yourself caught in a riptide, the inclination is to try and struggle back to shore against the current. That's how you end up drowning. If you recognize a force is pulling you, let it. Tread water as it drags you where it will. The currents will eventually change or subside, and you can return to shore. Even if you're pulled a mile from where you entered, that's okay; just walk back.

What does that mean in more practical terms? You now know that the source of your anxiety is an "I don't want to be here" thought, so reflect on how that process plays out in your present moment. When stress and anxiety escalate, your lizard brain jumps into the fray without waiting to see if the neocortex is following. Kick your neocortex into the game to inject some logical thinking. Recognize and acknowledge that you are feeling anxious. Identify that your stress response is kicking in, even if it's at a reduced level of intensity. Be aware that this automatic response is initiated by an unconscious thought of "I don't want to be here." You can complete this assessment in an instant. If you're at work and think you don't have time for reflection, you don't need more than a moment to detect that you're feeling anxious, that your fight-or-flight reflex is generating a non-helpful reaction, and that there is no inherent danger. You may not conclude this situation with a "win," but frame it as a learning opportunity. You know what happened and can pinpoint why by reflecting on the circumstance and possible triggers. Recognize that it happened, accept it, and commit to learning from it in the following day's reflection.

With Martina Hingis, the negative momentum driven by her stress and anxiety resulted in her losing the French Open. Okay, that's one match. What could she have learned from the situation to come back stronger? When failures happen, and our anxiety wins the day, reframe those situations from failures to teachable moments, offering vital insights to leverage in the next situation. If you freeze up in a meeting with an executive, you might reflect to yourself, "Okay, I didn't know how to respond in that meeting when our group VP questioned me. What could I do differently next time? When I'm in another meeting with that executive, I will anticipate areas of push-back and plan out three relevant responses that are generic enough to be leveraged across a range of questions. "

There is also a reversal of the "do nothing" strategy, which is (surprise) to "do something," anything really. At times, anxiety can leave us paralyzed. The work requests are piling up, and we find ourselves frozen, unable to start on any of the tasks as the stress consumes us. Or perhaps we recognize the enormity of the job at hand. A visual scan of our home confirms that it will take 8 hours to clean what's become a disaster area. We choose to do nothing because we'll never find a free 8 hours to complete the job. If you're overwhelmed by the enormity of what's before you, leverage the 80/20 rule and focus on the 20 percent of tasks that will make the most significant impact. If your house is a mess, picking up the loose items and vacuuming the carpet will make a meaningful difference, even if you can't wash the windows and the floor.

Are you feeling run down and tired? The temptation will be to lie down on the couch, making yourself feel even more tired and unaccomplished for the day. Instead, take the opposite action of your inclination to lay on the couch and get outside for a walk or run. You'll be surprised how expending energy actually serves to generate a surge of energy in return. Are you watching your kids play at a playground and bored out of your mind? Force yourself to get up and engage with them in play. As you feel the negative thoughts building and realize that you're doing nothing from fear or lack of motivation, force yourself to engage with what's in front of you and watch how it alters your mood.

If you sit there inactive, passively taking it all in, that idleness will invite rumination. When you catch yourself repeating negative thoughts, actively engage in another activity that requires your conscious attention and can displace the negativity cycle. Are you sitting at the beach knowing that you should be enjoying a day with your family and appreciating the beautiful surroundings, yet you just keep going over the challenges you face at work or home as you recline on a chair? Do something instead to occupy your conscious thought. Engage your spouse in a meaningful conversation. Get up off the beach chair and splash around with your kids. Get everyone to take a walk down the beach for some ice cream. Remember how we discussed the brain's inability to multitask as a limitation? By engaging in other actions and activities, we're using our inability to multitask to our advantage as we displace the negative thoughts.

As we reviewed in Chapter 4, "*Power in Presence*," engaging instead of observing is a highly effective proactive tool to head off anxiety, stress, and other negative emotions before they manifest. In addition, engaging in a new, focused task is a powerful tactic to break us out of the cycle when we begin to ruminate and descend into an anxiety spiral. The new activity stops the momentum as we make it impossible for our brain to continue its rehashing of the negatives. As mentioned in the timeout section, changing our behavior represents the reversal of the CBT progression from thoughts to feelings to actions, focusing instead on choosing your actions to influence your feelings and thoughts. Leverage the benefits of cognitive dissonance, that distressed state when our thoughts conflict with our actions, where our brain will seek to bring harmony between the two.

When we consciously choose a positive action and commit to it, our brain won't have any choice but to give in and replace the harmful thoughts with ones that better match our current behavior.

Putting it all Together

In the 1974 fight dubbed the "Rumble in the Jungle," Muhammad Ali faced off against George Foreman in perhaps the greatest fight of his career and arguably the best fight in boxing history. Going into the bout, Ali was the older former champion, having been stripped of the heavyweight title and serving a more than three-year ban from boxing for his refusal to join the U.S. Army through the draft in 1967. Foreman, on the other hand, looked to be an unstoppable force. He was seven years younger than Ali, at 25, and came in as the undefeated champion, having recently destroyed Joe Frazier and Ken Norton, the only two men to have beaten Ali.

Ali was known for his evasive style in the ring, counterpunching as he danced away from opponents. Everyone believed Ali would do the same against Foreman, spending the fight running from the younger and more powerful fighter. Despite his past conventions, in the opening round, Ali came out and, instead of running, went toe-to-toe with Foreman as he attacked the younger man with powerful blows. Foreman, likely stunned by the tactic, took some punishment early on but came back in the round to deliver potent shots of his own and end the round with momentum.[10]

In the 2nd round, Ali changed tactics and neither danced around nor stood toe-to-toe with Foreman. Instead, his strategy seemed to be to do *nothing*. Ali literally began leaning back onto the ropes, allowing Foreman to deliver powerful punches unchallenged. But Ali covered up, as the announcers observed that most of Foreman's blows weren't scoring any points as they were absorbed by Ali's arms or missed the mark altogether.

Some of Foreman's punches broke through Ali's defenses, but Ali quickly tied Foreman up with his arms and leaned his weight on the younger man while pushing down on his head. During these tie-ups, Ali appears to be screaming things at Foreman. As the round progresses, Ali, picking his moments, effectively counter-punches and lands several straight shots to Foreman's head, but he does so while still from his position leaning on the ropes. Round two ends up being a close contest. As the men return to their corners after the round, Foreman sits on his stool, visibly gasping for breath.

Rounds three and four follow a similar pattern as Ali's strategy becomes clear. None of Foreman's fights in recent years had gone past the third round, as he ended most quickly by knockout. Foreman wasn't used to going into the deeper rounds, and Ali tried to wear him down as he prolonged the fight. As Ali continued to yell at Foreman, taunting him with claims like, "You can't hurt me!" it became clear that Ali was baiting Foreman to keep attacking with all his force.

While rounds two, three, and four saw Ali regularly counter punching from his position on the ropes, he took the strategy even further in the fifth round. Ali spends the first 75% of the round leaning back on the ropes, protecting himself, all while taunting Foreman to keep hitting him. He allows Foreman to throw huge punches while he covers up, making little attempt to respond. The announcers believe Ali is tired and beginning to take punishment. Then, in the twilight of the round, Ali erupts with a flurry of activity that leaves Foreman dazed. This pattern then continues for the next few rounds, with Ali laying back until the later stages of each. As round seven begins, Ali walks straight to the ropes and leans back against them without even trying to engage first. He leans and waits for Foreman to attack.

In several breaks between previous rounds, Ali stood up and incited the crowd, as they chanted repeatedly, "Ali Bomaye!" which means "Ali, kill him!" The break after the seventh round is handled differently. Ali sits in his corner and begins breathing deeply, slowly, and intentionally. Round eight looks a lot like round seven, with Ali leaning back against the ropes, allowing Foreman to throw more barrages of punches, but those punches are slowing down. It appears the round will end there without Ali doing much of anything in response, but with just 15 seconds remaining, Ali flips their positions and faces Foreman from the center of the ring. He delivers a flurry of punches, and Foreman goes down with only seconds remaining in the round. The referee counts out Foreman, and Ali improbably wins by knockout. Pandemonium ensues in the Zaire stadium as fans go wild with exuberance and people flood the ring. Ali won the heavyweight championship, and in stunning fashion.

***

What can we learn from Ali's fight against Foreman? Foreman is like the overwhelming momentum of our anxiety. Ali attempts to face this unyielding force in the first round, taking Foreman head-on. While his direct tactic is valiant and results in initial success, Foreman's power and relentless attacks are too overwhelming for Ali to continue in this strategy. At the timeout between rounds, Ali takes the opportunity to assess the situation and changes his tactics. He comes out in round two and implements his "do nothing" strategy, which he would later dub the "rope a dope." Ali recognizes that running will tire *him* out and that he can't survive a firefight, so he lies back and protects himself, goading Foreman to expend his energy while Ali bides his time.

During the fight, Ali can be seen and heard screaming at Foreman repeatedly. Ali tells Foreman he can't hurt Ali, provokes him to throw more punches, and mocks his power. These acts are Ali's self-talk and inner thoughts being outwardly proclaimed at the force trying to destroy him. Ali repeated these assertions so many times during the fight that he no-doubt believed them. As his strategy required absorbing an incredible number of punches from his formidable opponent, Ali could have started to spiral during those long minutes, reflecting on the pain and punishment he was taking. Instead, he kept his mind engaged and his thoughts focused, repeatedly shouting his declarations, leaving no space for negative thoughts to build.

At a timeout after the seventh round, Ali takes the opportunity for intentional, deep, and calming breaths to prepare him for what would be his final round of punishment. After laying back idly for almost the entirety of the eighth round, Ali suddenly springs into action to end the fight in seconds. While Ali's key tactic was doing nothing as Foreman expended all his energy, Ali picked key moments to engage himself in the contest.

In the same way, anxiety is a powerful force that can build seemingly unstoppable momentum, but if we stop feeding it through our negative thoughts, it will run out of steam. While Ali pulled off the improbable victory that day, not every one of *our* fights with anxiety will end in triumph, but each day represents only a single battle. The next day, we can turn the page, reset physically and mentally, and plan adjustments to our strategy.

George Foreman, the loser in the fight, demonstrated this capacity to move on from his defeat. Though it took him time to appreciate, he eventually recognized that the fight was over. He had lost, and nothing would change that. He shared in an interview in 1981, "I had to look him in the eye and say, 'I lost. He beat me.' Before that, I had nothing but revenge and hate on my mind, but from then on, it was clear. I'll never be able to win that match, so I had to let it go."[11] Foreman let the loss go, and Ali became one of Foreman's closest friends until Ali passed.

The final lesson from the great fight is that our preparation dictates our capacity to meet and conquer our biggest challenges. Muhammad Ali's improbable victory didn't happen by accident. His ability to withstand the barrage of body blows he faced surprised the announcers, but he had completed an intense abdominal exercise regimen leading up to the fight. His continual verbal provocations of Foreman in the ring weren't improv comedy; they were calculated tactics to initiate Foreman's attacks. His strategic pivot at the end of the first round wasn't determined on the fly; it was part of a brilliant strategy laid out in advance. His moves were planned, and he entered the fight having prepared his body and mind for the punishment he knew was ahead.

If we want not just to survive the next wave of anxious thoughts that threaten to overtake us but instead to conquer them, it requires hard work, discipline, and strategic planning. If we don't proactively plan the right thoughts, practice their reinforcement, and prepare our minds for when the wrong ones appear, we can't expect to stand victorious when our negative thoughts manifest, and anxiety gains momentum. Ali stated, reflecting on the work required to succeed, "I hated every minute of training, but I said, 'Don't quit. Suffer now and live the rest of your life as a champion.'"[12]

Chapter Eight

It Will Be Hard, But We Can Make It Easy

There is a story in the Bible in the book of First Kings, Chapter 18, where God's prophet Elijah accomplishes more improbable feats in a single day than most great figures can claim from an entire lifetime. In this supercharged 24 hours, Elijah calls down fire from heaven to consume an immense sacrifice, he brings about a rainstorm through his prayer to end a great drought, and, perhaps most miraculously, he runs a distance of 16 miles, outpacing the king of Israel's chariot the entire way. In completing these three miracles, Elijah's version of a triathlon puts today's most challenging Ironman competitions to shame. While conducting these acts, Elijah faced down a king and hundreds of religious leaders who wanted him dead. He stood defiantly against these adversaries with great faith, confidence, and emotional strength.

Then, everything changed. A mere one chapter later, after having emerged victorious in a struggle against these powerful men, Elijah encounters the king of Israel's wife, Jezebel. Hearing about Elijah's exploits and filled with rage, Jezebel threatens to kill Elijah. No problem, right? Elijah just stood tall against hundreds who wanted the same outcome, including the king. A threat from the king's wife seems small by comparison. Yet upon hearing the threat, Elijah takes off running for the wilderness. He finds refuge under a tree where he prays to die, pleading with God, "I have had enough, Lord. Take my life, for I am no better than my ancestors who have already died."[1]

What happened to the marathon-running, fire-from-heaven-calling, drought-breaking champion from the previous chapter? In response to Elijah's prayer, God could have answered directly, with appeals to logic and reason. He could have reminded Elijah of the miracles He had just empowered Elijah to complete. God could have recounted all the tests and trials He had brought Elijah through over the years. He could have told Elijah that He wouldn't have brought him this far, only to let him fall at the hands of Jezebel now. Instead, God decides not to address Elijah's pleas for the end at all. Rather than reasoning with Elijah, God sends an angel to bring Elijah food and water, not once but twice, which Elijah enjoys between restorative naps. Feeling revived, Elijah continues his great journey, traveling 40 days and nights to Mount Sinai to meet with God.

What was the difference between the man who was one day filled with power and mental strength and the one who experienced a mental breakdown the next day? Hunger, thirst, and exhaustion. It's hard to keep focused on positive thoughts when we're tired, hungry, or thirsty. If those needs are unfulfilled for too long (which, in my case, is missing a single meal), it's a challenge to think about anything else. We will also struggle to be in the right mental state when other, higher-order needs aren't met. For instance, if we haven't done our favorite activities in a long time, if it's been too long since we accomplished something we're proud of, or if we haven't had meaningful connections with our friends and family. Being intentional in fulfilling these different levels of needs can turn establishing mental strength from "mission impossible" to a lasting personal attribute.

Taking Care of the Essentials

I'll state the obvious but then explore why it's easier said than done: when you're hungry, eat; when you're thirsty, hydrate; and when you're exhausted, prioritize a good night's sleep. This is not quite groundbreaking advice, but if we're not careful, we will miss that there are basic needs we're putting off and that their deferral adversely affects our mental state and interactions with others.

At work, I have regular one-on-one meetings with my teammates. The interactions are usually good; we share some of what's going on in our lives and then get into the work topics. Yet, I've had periods when the dynamics were off. The discussions felt more challenging than needed, and I knew both sides weren't particularly enjoying them. These were good people, and the work was engaging, so what was going on?

I realized my struggles coincided with meeting times when I tended to get hungry. Our brain cells are fed by glucose. When our blood sugar drops, that inhibits the optimal functioning of the brain and, therefore, our thinking. Hunger releases different hormones into our bodies, such as ghrelin, known as the "hunger hormone." Ghrelin is produced in the stomach, and the hunger signal is transmitted to our brain. The hormone may also directly impact our moods. Beyond ghrelin, hunger can produce epinephrine or adrenaline, which is associated with our stress response. This stress can add to both feelings of anxiety and aggression. In other words, "hanger," the state of getting angry when hungry, is real.[2] But eating doesn't just keep us from generating negative feelings and stress; it also contributes to our happiness. Eating something we enjoy can release dopamine and endorphins, hormones that make us feel good. If we can simultaneously cut off negative emotions while building positive ones, those are two strong votes favoring coupling one-on-one meetings and snack time.

I started putting food within reach for all my meetings. I prioritized eating during the sessions rather than outside them to avoid over-eating. All good things have their detractors, and some people may consider eating a protein bar on a video call a break in etiquette. For me, the benefits of better interactions and an improved mood are well worth the potential etiquette violation. Also, I try to eat relatively video-appropriate things, so I'll typically wait to gnaw on a chicken leg until the call concludes. If you're overly concerned with the optics of chewing in a meeting, have a smoothie instead and sip it during the discussion. Try to keep the camera on, as video is better for presence and connection than audio alone. The same practice can apply whether you're remote or in person, and I actually find it easier to eat during in-person meetings, as you don't have a camera right in your face.

With pangs of hunger pacified and endorphins flowing through me, staying fully present and engaged in the conversations became effortless. Changing my eating habits had a surprisingly significant impact on re-establishing satisfaction and fun in these interactions (I suspect both for me and my meeting counterparts). In the same way I discovered that *I* was the source of the challenges with my boss described in Chapter 6, "*The Higher Call*," I once again found that the fault for a difficult work interaction didn't lie with someone else; the accountability and the power to change the dynamic was with me.

Outside of work, these same scenarios were playing out at home. During the bedtime routine with my kids, when I help them bathe, get dressed, brush their teeth, and read them books, I found myself getting irritable and anticipating when I could go back downstairs for a nightly snack. Rather than focusing on being present and appreciating that I was "where I wanted to be," I was looking past those moments to enjoy something far less meaningful.

I had created an environment where the snack served as a reward for completing my job, the bedtime routine. I had unconsciously framed the bedtime process as a chore and its completion as my goal. Yet the reality is that the bedtime routine and time with my kids should have been the best part of my day. Once I was done putting them to bed and was downstairs eating, I would inevitably wish I hadn't rushed through the process. It feels silly how long I stayed in this suboptimal pattern. Thankfully, I eventually made the practical decision to bring up the food I wanted and eat while I completed the bedtime duties. Sure, bringing up my snacks caused other challenges, like my kids wanting me to share with them after brushing their teeth. However, that was easier to manage now that my hunger was satisfied, and I wasn't holding out on some gratification until after the bedtime routine was completed. I could linger with them a little longer and enjoy it. "You want one more story? Great, me too." Did my little princess daughter want me to sit with her for another minute? Fantastic, because I didn't want to be anywhere else.

Do you think I'm just weird about my eating habits and that I'm overstating the relationship between food and our mental wellbeing? The truth is I may not be making the case strongly enough, as a well-timed snack break has been demonstrated to impact decisions of freedom itself. In 2011, a team that included a cognitive neuroscience PhD and a professor at Columbia Business School published a research paper titled "Extraneous Factors in Judicial Decisions."[3] The team analyzed over 1,000 parole decisions made by a group of Israeli judges spanning ten months. They found that the time of the day significantly impacted the potential for parole to be granted. During parts of the day, about 65% of cases were granted parole. Those levels then consistently fell, reaching a point where almost none of the cases concluded with a favorable ruling. What was causing the variability at different periods?

The team found the delineating factor was when the judges had a break for a snack or lunch. They were far more lenient right after the break, with the 65% favorability rate in their rulings. The further they got from the break, the closer to 0% those rates became. The findings indicate that factors that should have no bearing on the cases themselves (such as the timing of lunch, the hunger level of the judge, and mental fatigue) can have an astronomical impact on decisions between freedom and continued imprisonment. The implication for me is that if I ever find myself in front of a judge, I will be sure to hand them a granola bar before pleading my case.

***

Sleep is another essential we should be intentional about. The link between sleep deprivation and stress is something we've all experienced firsthand. Writing this book has taken many long nights alongside a full-time job and raising young kids. On several occasions, I realized the next day that I was tired and feeling especially vulnerable to even moderate stressors. Depriving my body of its required rest served to stack the deck against me, making it easier for unhelpful thoughts to enter my psyche.

Yet sleep isn't just a deterrent to stressful thinking or a bad mood. Sleep is when we get stronger, both physically and mentally. If you work out during the day, sleep is when your muscles are repaired, and you grow new tissue. The same process applies to mental strength, as sleep is vital in building the neural pathways we discussed previously. As we intentionally practice a new activity, including cultivating new thought patterns, many neurons fire that aren't required to complete that task. The correct path is obscured by fog. As we sleep, the essential neural pathways needed to complete a specific task are reinforced. When we attempt to proactively introduce the right thoughts as we approach a potentially stressful situation, we'll find the process difficult and awkward the first time. However, if we follow practice with a good night's sleep, approaching the potentially stressful situation with the right mindset will come more naturally the next time.[4]

The right amount of sleep will differ for everyone. Is 6 hours sufficient? That's fine, but be careful you're not fooling yourself, as many studies have demonstrated boosts in performance when increasing sleep duration.[5,6] It's okay if you need 9 hours of sleep to feel at your best. Plenty of elite athletes sleep for above-average periods. Quarterback Tom Brady goes to bed at 8:30 p.m.[7] Basketball star Lebron James prioritizes 10 hours of sleep per night.[8] Olympic gymnast Simone Biles sleeps 8 hours, supplemented by daytime naps after training sessions.[9] Those tendencies may be expected of professional athletes who push their bodies to their limits during waking hours. However, many elite academics who rely on mental rather than physical strength have prioritized sleep similarly. Albert Einstein represents possibly the greatest mind of modern times. His thought experiments transformed our understanding of the physical world and shaped innumerable technological advances. He is said to have regularly slept 10 hours a night, in addition to frequent naps.[10]

Our starting point for each day is the conclusion of sleep from the night before. A big part of establishing positive momentum is starting strong. Beginning the day feeling rested provides an initial boost to jump-start positive momentum that builds through the day. It's best to be proactive in getting enough sleep instead of waking up to discover we've cut ourselves short.

However, if we wake up and realize we've missed out on a good night's sleep, it's over; don't dwell on it. Our thoughts are our most powerful tool. Don't perpetuate negative momentum by regretting the sleep you didn't get the night before. Recognize that you have the rest and strength needed to succeed on this day. Tonight, you can prioritize getting optimal rest for the next day.

***

Throughout the book, we've focused on how our thoughts are the source of our feelings and actions. Yet now we're discussing how various hormones can impact our mood and behaviors, introducing stress, aggression, or, on the flip side, happiness. So which is it? Do our thoughts drive our feelings and behaviors, or are the hormones the real driver? The answer is that hormones significantly influence our mental state, but they are not the source.

The release of hormones is triggered by different factors, sometimes by our thoughts and other times by our actions. For example, we've identified that the source of a "fight-or-flight" response is the thought, "I don't want to be here." That fight-or-flight system triggers the release of stress hormones like adrenaline and cortisol. The release of these hormones isn't the *source* of our stress and state of high alert; it is a *response* to that stress and prepares our bodies to deal with it. The "I don't want to be here" thought drives the hormone release and the subsequent feelings. If we can condition different thoughts, we will avoid releasing these hormones, or we will release different, more helpful ones.

In addition, we can take actions that facilitate both the release of hormones and the reduction of hormone levels. We've discussed how eating can release different hormones that make us happy. Sleep and intentional breathing can serve to reduce stress hormones. Exercise releases endorphins to make us feel good. Serotonin, the ultimate mood regulator, can help fight off anxiety and depression. Serotonin levels can be boosted through exercise, a healthy diet, and exposure to sunlight.

Scientists have identified over 50 hormones in the human body.[11] These hormones are produced by glands that occupy our brains and other bodily regions. The glands send signals to the cell receptors of our organs, including our brains, influencing how they respond. This process and network are called the endocrine system. The endocrine system is responsible for many bodily processes, like growth and development, metabolism, and the sleep-wake cycle, but it also plays a significant role in shaping our moods.

The net effect is that these naturally created chemicals or drugs are constantly pumped through our bodies. All these hormones serve a valuable purpose, including those I've described as having negative implications. Adrenaline and cortisol are essential hormones that we need a boost of when taking on many physical activities. However, those same hormones can be counterproductive when our brains misinterpret their need.

Consider a trip to the dentist. The dentist may share that you have a cavity and need a filling. Before the procedure, they say you'll need an injection of the numbing medicine Novocain to dull any pain from the required tooth drilling. But what if you got that shot of Novocain, and then the doctor decided that instead of giving you a filling, you just needed your teeth brushed? They give you a thorough brushing and send you on your way. You have clean teeth, but you also experience a temporary loss of feeling in your face from the numbing medicine. It would be pretty frustrating to spend the next few hours slurring your words and drooling on yourself when there was no need for it. In the same way, we don't want to allow the release of these hormones that mess with our physiology when there isn't a practical purpose.

Given these hormones serve as powerful influencers on our moods and feelings, we want to aid in their operation, enabling them to be deployed when needed and helpful. The body will handle this task on autopilot, but we can step in and impact its operation with our conscious thoughts and actions.

As we've discussed, the relationship between our thoughts, feelings, and actions can be bidirectional. When our thoughts shape our feelings, the release of hormones follows the thoughts and can be controlled by changing them. When the flow is reversed, and our actions impact our feelings, the release of hormones follows the actions. If we want to naturally harness the power of these chemicals pumping through our bodies, then we need to practice the right behaviors, which we instill as habits so that they stick.

Establishing the Right Habits

My wife, Suzy, calls me an extremist. She's not wrong, and while I'm not quite sure she means it as a compliment, I see significant benefits in going far beyond the average. What does average get us? An average diet and activity level (especially in the United States) leaves us susceptible to health problems. An average job and salary may mean we can't have abundance or give abundantly. An average marriage has a dangerously high potential for ending in divorce. An average relationship with our kids puts them at risk of being influenced more by social media than by our values. Average is 50%, and if we settle for 50%, we leave the other 50% on the table. That's a lot to give up. Our outputs are a reflection of our inputs. If we don't want to settle for average, we need to establish behaviors that are exceptional. Then, we need to make those behaviors repeatable by ingraining them as habits.

Since the time of my panic attack almost a decade ago, I've systematically developed a set of habits that, while none are revolutionary, are each uncommon in today's Western culture. These habits have served to strengthen my mind and body. While *developing* these habits was not easy, *practicing* them has become not only easy but enjoyable. The implication is greater ease in staving off negative feelings and generating positive thoughts that stick.

I'll briefly describe my personal habits but then spend more time on how you can cultivate your habits of choice, as the "right" habits for you will likely differ from the ones I practice. The habits I've focused on developing since the peak of my anxiety include exercise, diet, cold showers, learning and development, and preparation.

My daily exercise regimen consists of a morning run of a few miles and another three-mile run later in the day, accompanied by a short but high-intensity workout where I cycle through strength training for every body part. I'm always looking for the small random acts of exercise I can tack on during the day as well. For instance, my kids' school playground has a rope I quickly climb daily when I drop them off. One day, this habit may land me in the principal's office, but for now, it's a risk worth taking. If I have an opportunity to add a physical activity or exercise in the evening, I take it. I'll complete at least the same activity level on the weekends, but usually more. I run and do strength training every day of the year. I've had periods where I have an injury, but I'll adjust with a replacement activity, like biking or swimming instead of running, rather than resting.

When it comes to eating, my diet isn't of the special name-brand variety but is closest to the paleo diet. I only eat vegetables, fruit, meat, beans, nuts, eggs, and a bit of sea salt. I don't eat grains, dairy, or consume any processed sugar. I drink only water and unsweetened coconut water after workouts. I don't have coffee, tea, juices, or alcohol. There are no "cheat days" with my diet.

For learning and development, my primary vehicle is books. For the past decade, I've been consuming all the books I could on topics such as anxiety and public speaking, as well as those covering business, economics, science, technology, biographies, and other nonfiction categories. If I'm struggling with something, recognize a deficiency in my knowledge, or find an emerging topic relevant to my work, I'll find a book (or multiple) on the subject. Whenever I'm engaged in an activity I can complete on autopilot (such as running, walking, doing the dishes, or cleaning up), I simultaneously listen to an audiobook on one of these topics. Then, I read from a digital book at night. Between reading at night and audiobooks, I'll go through three to four books per month.

The cold shower habit is pretty self-explanatory; instead of turning the nozzle to the "H," I keep the dial right there at the "C" for "Cold." Fortunately, I've never encountered a situation where my family has used up all the cold water.

I know the cold showers sound appealing, but it's possible you will think that "fun" is conspicuously absent from my habit list. Now, I haven't detailed every activity. I don't watch much TV, but I love watching movies with my kids. My fitness regimen often includes sports or games rather than exclusively "working out." For instance, I regularly play pickleball with my wife and friends.

It's not a stretch to frame movies and games as fun, but I can honestly state that I also genuinely enjoy each of the daily habits I mentioned. Why do I not have a "rest day" from exercise? Because I *like* to exercise. On the weekends, I will do more of what I enjoy, not less. In the same way, I don't need a "cheat day" in my diet because I love the foods I eat. Eating a mix of fresh vegetables, chicken, and avocado, with lemon juice and sea salt, is much more appealing than the sandwiches I used to eat for lunch with processed deli meat.

Getting your habits to a point of enjoyment is critical, as that is a crucial element of making them stick. If you've established a weekday-only habit and the weekend is your "reward" to break from that routine, you will always draw against finite stores of willpower. Those cold showers? I've come to enjoy the rush from the cold water, which feels particularly good after working up a sweat.

Were these activities all enjoyable when I started each practice? No, because my body and mind were conditioned to enjoy other options. What have I done? I've reset my expectations of what these activities should entail and how they should be characterized. For instance, we're trained to believe that bathing should only be done in warm or hot water. Why is that? If we go to the beach, we're happy to jump in the cold ocean and find it refreshing. You could have that same feeling of refreshment every time you shower.

Having genuine enjoyment for these activities does not mean I bounce out of bed every morning, skipping down the stairs to my run. I'll often need reminding and reinforcement that what I am about to do, I want to do. However, that requirement for reinforcement is true of many other good and meaningful things in our lives.

What do all these habits do? They all release hormones into our bodies that can boost our mood while reducing stress and anxiety. We've covered the hormones connected to food and exercise. With reading, the primary benefit will be the knowledge you gain and the power of that knowledge. In addition, the act of reading itself can release dopamine, serotonin, and endorphins that make you feel good, as well as reduce the stress hormone cortisol. Cold water exposure produces the feel-good hormones of endorphins, serotonin, and dopamine and releases stress hormones, including cortisol and norepinephrine. Remember, those hormones aren't inherently bad. When we experience a stressor like cold water, it's good for the heart to work harder and our blood pressure to rise to maintain our core temperature.

In fact, exposing ourselves to these healthy stressors builds our mental toughness and our resilience to stress. Neuroscientist and Stanford Professor Andrew Huberman described in a 2022 newsletter on his website, that when we choose to step into a stressful environment, such as cold exposure, we are training our brains to exert control over stressful situations.[12] When we later encounter stressful circumstances that we haven't chosen, our practice kicks in, and we are better equipped to deal with the stress. The same benefit applies to exercise, as the stress we voluntarily introduce through physical activity conditions the body to better cope with non-voluntary forms of stress.

An entertaining (as well as gruesome) study conducted in 2020 and published in the Journal of Neuroscience by the research team Tillage, Wilson, Liles, Holmes, and Weinshenker explored the relationship between voluntary stress and resilience.[13] The researchers took two groups of mice and made one group work out for three weeks by introducing running wheels, while the other group got to lounge around all day in their cages that were not equipped with mice treadmills. The workout mice ran between 6 and 10 miles per day, with an interesting peripheral finding being that female mice ran significantly more than the males (win one for the ladies). After three weeks, the researchers introduced stress to both groups by shocking their feet and analyzed how they responded, including their subsequent ability to conduct different tasks.

The stressed mice who had been working out demonstrated significantly higher resilience compared with the sedentary mice. When analyzing the "freeze" response to the shocks, a fear response when the animals stopped moving, measured in seconds, the exercise mice shook off the shocks, freezing, on average, for only 10 to 15 seconds. On the other hand, the sedentary mice froze up for more than a full minute on average. Remember, the fight-or-flight response is often called "fight, flight, or freeze." Regular exercise made the mice far more resilient to succumbing to a "fight, flight, or freeze" reaction.

Oh, what about the gruesome aspect of the study that I mentioned? While many other studies have demonstrated a similar connection between exercise and mental strength, this study was in search of the specific molecular structures in the brain associated with this type of resilience. Tragically, to arrive at their conclusions, the researchers decapitated the mice after the behavioral analysis so they could study their brains. Now it's clear why I'm citing a study conducted on mice instead of people.

Returning to our discussion of habits, all these example activities (diet, reading, exercise, and cold exposure) deploy the natural resources we have available to give us the best chance of mental well-being during the day. They pull the levers within our control to stack the deck in our favor. Even better, certain habits where we voluntarily introduce stressors, like exercise and cold exposure, offer the added benefit of conditioning our minds to build resilience and respond better to stressful situations in the future.

When it comes to our diet, the most important factor is getting the proper nutrition. What we put in our bodies impacts our physical and mental well-being. Has anyone ever finished half a greasy pizza and said, "I feel amazing and am going to go run a marathon." No, you're more likely to feel on the verge of a coma after a meal like that. There are plenty of great resources that can further inform you of the benefits of proper nutrition. So instead of talking about the advantages of vegetables over grease, I'm going to indulge in a little speculative research that has some rough edges but may change the way you think about your diet, as well as explain why it's so hard to change. While still emerging and yet to offer definitive conclusions, this field of study presents a fascinating perspective on how the food we eat impacts our cognition.

What's not under debate is that we live alongside billions of microorganisms or microbes. These tiny living organisms inhabit our skin, mouths, and even our bodies. Those who call our insides their home are collectively called the human microbiota, with the greatest concentration in our gut. Think you'd rather go through life without them? You'd have a hard time, as you depend on your microbiota for your health and well-being. They play essential functions in breathing, digestion, the immune system, and even hormone regulation, impacting our moods and mental health.

We reviewed previously how the "hunger hormone," ghrelin, is released by our stomach and signals to the brain that we're hungry. A connection pathway between our stomach (and, more broadly, the gastrointestinal system or "gut") and the brain, called the gut-brain axis, makes this line of communication possible. Our microbiota are common callers on this communication line, regularly sending and influencing signals to the brain. The Cleveland Clinic notes on its website, "Certain bacteria actually produce or stimulate the production of neurotransmitters (like serotonin) that send chemical signals to your brain."[14] What's the implication? The gut microbes, these separate living entities, send signals to our brains that, while not controlling us, have significant influence over our feelings and behaviors.

There are good microbes that support our health, well-being, and digestion, and there are harmful microbes, known as pathogenic bacteria, which can release toxins, inhibit the absorption of nutrients, and allow infections to enter our bloodstream. The Cleveland Clinic notes that different microbes "prefer" or "favor" different foods. The helpful microbes feed off various plant fibers and even require them for survival, while studies suggest that many pathogenic or "bad" microbes thrive on processed foods and processed sugar.

As these are living organisms, if we don't feed them what they need for survival, they'll die off. If we give them what they need, they'll thrive and multiply. A diet based on fast-food cheeseburgers and fries will support a colony of unhelpful bacteria. If we eat lots of fruits and vegetables, we nurture a community of beneficial gut microbes. A healthy microbiota composition is critical to our physical and mental health.

Elaine Hsiao, a Professor in Biological Sciences at UCLA, is doing pioneering research in the field. She notes, "More and more research is revealing that the gut microbiome can influence the brain and behavior across a variety of different animals."[15] While causal relationships are yet to be definitively established, do you want the potential for your brain to be controlled by pathogenic, fast-food-addicted organisms?

This relationship between our mental state and microbiota also indicates why it's so hard to change our diets and why we feel addicted to certain foods. We're not just fighting our own preferences and addictions; we're dealing with those of our tiny friends as well. If particular diets sustain different classes of microbes, and those microbes can signal the brain with hormones like serotonin, what's the implication? It means that feeding our fast-food-loving microbes sends our brain pleasure signals that make us want to continue eating those foods. Imagine a tiny but vast army of organisms in our guts, demanding we satisfy their need for McDonald's.

As we change our diet, we change the microbiota composition. These changes can happen quickly, which Rachel Carmody, a Harvard Assistant Professor of Evolutionary Biology and principal investigator of the department's Nutritional and Microbial Ecology Lab, demonstrated in her 2021 research. Her study swapped the diets of domesticated dogs and wolves, feeding the dogs raw meat and the wolves processed dog food. Carmody found that the microbial makeup of the animals quickly shifted, with significant changes measured in as little as 24 hours. The dogs began to cultivate a microbe composition that resembled that of wolves, with the wolves' microbe population resembling that of dogs.[16] While changes to the microbiota makeup can happen quickly, the lasting nature of those changes remains a topic of study.

I've eaten semi-healthy since adulthood, but my willpower always wanes towards the end of the day. For years, at night, I would find myself sitting on the couch, eating ice cream directly from the carton or having a third of a container of baked goods. The microbes in my gut were sustained by those processed foods high in fat and processed sugars. I still have plenty of food cravings, but now they are for date and nut bars and fruit and nut smoothies.

While it took time to shift my habits and for my cravings to adjust, I now have zero desire for the unhealthy foods I used to eat. The absence of those cravings isn't for lack of availability, as my kids would stage a violent revolt if I forced my diet upon them (their microbes are quite passionate). So ice cream, cookies, and candy are always present in our house. A crucial component of making my healthy diet stick, which I've now practiced for years, was cutting off the consumption of the unhealthy foods totally and without exception. I showed no mercy, starving out every last one of those milkshake-loving microbes.

***

Now, let's explore how we establish our chosen habits. In his book *Atomic Habits*, James Clear describes the habit loop, which outlines how habits originate with a cue or trigger, resulting in a craving, eliciting a response, and concluding with a reward.[17] Clear's 'four laws of behavior change' connect with the habit loop's four steps. To create good habits, we should make them obvious (the cue), attractive (the craving), easy (the response), and satisfying (the reward).

Take the example of my morning run. When the alarm goes off in the morning, that's my cue that it's time to get up and run. I don't have to make any conscious decisions or tradeoffs because that's what I do every day when I wake up. To make a habit attractive, Clear advocates pairing activities we *want* to do with those we *need* to do. Even if it's not always fun to start the run, I can anticipate the good feelings that accompany being outside, getting into a rhythm, and the sense of accomplishment when I'm done. To make it easy, I avoid driving to a gym or establishing multiple preparation steps in advance. When my running shoes are on, I step out my front door and begin. To make it satisfying, beyond the good feelings I will have from the sense of accomplishment and the release of endorphins, I reward myself in a more tangible way with a coconut water when I'm done. Being intentional about those four steps allows us to establish a good habit.

To stop a bad habit, we must first identify the same steps in the loop. The response or the behavior is always clear, but it's often not obvious what cue or trigger initiates the loop. For instance, feeling stressed can be a trigger to initiate overeating, smoking, or irritability, but the critical piece of the puzzle is identifying the stress trigger. Once we detect the steps in our bad habit loop, we can work to remove the harmful practice. Clear's advice is to apply the inversion of the four laws of behavior change, making the behavior invisible, unattractive, difficult, and unsatisfying.

Taking the example of kicking my ice cream and baked goods nightly habit, I may not have removed all those items from the house to achieve the "invisibility" principle. However, I stopped buying them for myself and communicated that intention to my wife and kids. Our ice cream and baked goods are now intended as a treat for the kids and framed as "not for me." It's a subtle change that relied on how I perceived the same items in our cupboard or freezer, but if you believe reframing won't be enough, go ahead and eat your kids' Oreos and see if there isn't hell to pay in return.

In making the habit unattractive, I focused on the nutritional value of the foods. I previously didn't think critically about how the foods I ate contributed to my physical and mental well-being. If I was hungry and wanted something, I ate it. Paying more attention to nutrition, I recognized that the ingredients in most ice creams and baked goods lack benefits beyond a momentary taste experience. Now, I did love the refreshing taste of ice cream and milkshakes. So, I fulfilled that sensation with a healthy alternative in frozen banana smoothies. Over time, I've conditioned my tastes to prefer these banana and nut concoctions to the overwhelming processed sugar in ice cream.

This practice of replacement is essential, as removing a bad habit will leave a void to be filled. Take up that space with an intentionally selected healthy habit. To make the bad habit of unhealthy night eating difficult, I initially focused on eating a lot of my replacement foods (date bars and fruit smoothies) earlier in the evening. Filling myself up, especially with foods that satisfied my craving for desserts and sugar after a meal, made it difficult for me to want to eat *anything* later, good or bad.

Finally, to make the habit unsatisfying, I had to exercise patience. For the first several weeks, processed desserts still seemed appealing. At the same time, my replacement foods were genuinely enjoyable. I knew that if I stayed committed, those foods could replace and eventually surpass the more momentary satisfaction I received from unhealthy choices.

Clear's practical steps offer a valuable tool, but I even more appreciate two of his other insights: focusing on identity-based habits and the system over outcomes. In focusing on our identity, we first decide the person we want to be and then cultivate the habits to support that identity. The approach parallels our discussion on cognitive dissonance. If you choose to believe you are not a confident person at work, your brain will be perfectly comfortable supporting the behaviors of non-confident people. Don't raise your hand, don't contribute in that meeting, and say you "don't have anything to add" when you're called to share an opinion. On the other hand, if you start telling yourself you *are* a confident person, you'll put your brain in an uncomfortable spot until you start acting like it.

Once you make that bold claim of the type of person you are, identify the behaviors that support that identity. If you've always said you're not a morning person, what do you do when your morning alarm goes off? You hit the snooze button. You lie in bed for 10 minutes, dreading the inevitability of taking off the blanket. You walk around with a "don't talk to me until I've had my morning coffee" attitude. Start telling yourself you *are* a morning person instead. Even better, tell *others* you're a morning person, which will solidify the perception and build accountability. What behaviors will support that assertion? A morning person would place their alarm clock on the other side of the room. A morning person would sign up for the 6 a.m. spin class. A morning person would be the first one in the office. Leverage the power of claiming the identity you want and shape your habits to support that identity.

To appreciate Clear's other lesson of focusing on the system rather than outcome-oriented goals, the all-time great former University of Alabama football coach, Nick Saban, presents a gold-standard example. As detailed in John Talty's book, *The Leadership Secrets of Nick Saban*, Saban focuses his players on what they call "the process."[18] While Saban's teams were perennial national championship contenders, the outcome of winning a national title was not the goal Saban fixated his team on. Instead, "the process" focused his players on not just each opponent but each individual play.

Alabama players were conditioned to direct their total concentration to their specific job at each moment in a practice, workout, or game. In this way, Saban's teams were often relentless, running up the score on lesser opponents when other teams would have pulled back. Saban was infamous for chewing out players and coaches for lapses in judgment, such as taking unnecessary penalties, even when the game's outcome was no longer in question.

The point was that his teams were trained to stay fully engaged and to deliver their best work during every individual part of the game and at every part of practice, for that matter. Each discrete act was expected to be performed to the best of their abilities. While they directed their concentration to individual steps rather than the larger goal of winning national titles, national titles were still the outcome of Saban's process. In a Division 1 setting with well over 100 teams vying to be the best, Saban's teams competed in 9 national championship games during his 17-year tenure with Alabama, winning 6.

Establishing my own process at work to prepare for stressful situations was critical to not only building myself back up from the low of the panic attack but also allowing me to surge ahead with strength and confidence. As a big part of my job is to deliver presentations, I would always practice in advance. The problem was that my practice was not structured. I might rehearse a presentation 20 times, but as I thought of better points to make or improved ways to deliver those points, the result was 20 different iterations of the same presentation, each only practiced a single time.

My anxiety grew as I realized that as the moment of truth grew closer, I didn't know what I was going to say or how I was going to say it. The outcome of every presentation, and even my career itself, felt like it was hanging in the balance until the presentation was completed. The act of someone just *asking* me to give a presentation filled me with an immediate sense of anxiety. Even *watching* someone else present would build anxiety in me as I pictured myself in their place. Why was this process so effortless for some while it was driving me to the edge?

As I started studying the presentation habits of outstanding presenters and speakers like Steve Jobs, Winston Churchill, and Martin Luther King Jr., I realized that their all-time great speeches and presentations, which seemed effortless, took immense preparation and leveraged highly structured planning habits. I honed my process by studying these prominent figures and many others. For important presentations, I would write out precisely what I planned to say word-for-word. I would establish my story "throughline" in advance and pay particular attention to my transition statements between different points or slides. Writing out my script allowed me to ideally frame how I wanted to represent my thoughts and viewpoints. I would then practice each part in small chunks, first reading the chunk and then rehearsing it out loud until I was comfortable. After completing each chunk, I would practice the entire presentation from start to finish, from memory. When the time to present came, I never read from the script, and I felt the freedom to deviate from it, as I knew my material and could adjust to the audience or situation in real-time.

I started to incorporate lessons from other fields as well. Patricia Ryan Madson's book, *Improv Wisdom*, taught me to trust that the right words would be there when it was my turn to speak.[19] Also, while I knew I had a script and planned points to make, my audience had no clue, so if I forgot a detail, I would just move on to the next one. You can operate with peace and confidence when you show up to a test, knowing you already have all the answers. That confidence builds with repetition. Audiences I previously felt compelled to prepare hours for, I now feel comfortable with light or no preparation.

Beyond the wisdom offered by habit experts like James Clear, I add another step, which is the one my wife highlighted at the start of the chapter: extremism. If I leave a foothold for the wrong habits to creep in, they will. If I justify the existence of bad habits when carried out in moderation, I haven't committed to their replacement. I'm just keeping the bad habit at bay, which is a temporary fix, always dependent on willpower. If we quit smoking except when we're stressed, we're still a smoker. We'll frame our habit as "I'm trying to quit." Even if you still smoke, tell everyone around you, "I'm not a smoker." What do non-smokers not do, ever? Smoke. There are no compromises.

Don't bargain with your bad or good habits. Declare those you either want or don't want as aligning with your identity and follow through with complete commitment. And if you aspire to make a change, just do it. I've spent too much time thinking about habits I'd like to establish or wishing for new habits instead of just trying them out. I spent years working at my desk, wishing I was more active. I did not need to change careers to make that happen. I simply needed to prioritize my time, stop wishing, and start experimenting. Do you have an idea for a new habit? Try it out today. Don't wait until tomorrow.

***

All the most essential lessons for shaping our habits are rooted in the foundation of our thoughts. Our thoughts about our identities, the framing of our habits as enjoyable, good, or harmful, and a mindset of "no compromises" are all beliefs we hold. What people see are the actions and the outcomes, but they are the byproduct of the thoughts we have and the internal decisions we make. Outsized success may seem effortless for a casual observer, but that is rarely the reality. What will look like an overnight success is typically just the tip of the iceberg. Nick Saban will be remembered as one of the greatest coaches of all time based on his success at the University of Alabama, which he turned around seemingly "overnight." Yet Saban developed his "process" during the over three decades of coaching he committed himself to *before* joining Alabama.

Establishing your desired habits may not be easy, but once you've instilled healthy habits and rooted out the bad ones, you've created an environment where shaping the right thoughts is easy. If you don't get the proper nutrition, or if you're sleep-deprived, or if you haven't done things that you genuinely enjoy, claiming "I want to be here" will likely be met with a vocal rebuttal in your head. Suppose instead that you feel refreshed from sufficient sleep, that you have the benefit of serotonin and endorphins pumping to your brain from good food and exercise, and that you've trained your body and your mind to rise to the challenges you'll face through the introduction of controlled and healthy stressors. With those factors in place, practicing an "I want to be here" mentality can feel both achievable and expected, even in the face of adversity.

The personal habits I've shared are optimized for my life and what I want to accomplish. Based on who *you* want to be, identify the unique habits that help you get there. While many of my example habits focus on discipline and reframing hard things as enjoyable, prioritize the leisure habits in your routine as well. The objective is to establish the habits that help you show up as your best in the most meaningful moments.

Winston Churchill was known for keeping an exhausting schedule, including consistent late-night war cabinet meetings followed by early mornings. He had the weight of a nation, and in many ways, the world, on his shoulders during World War

II. Yet during those times, he still prioritized the things that would make him feel good physically and mentally. He took meetings from his bed in the morning. He ate fried bacon and eggs for breakfast. He drank alcohol throughout the day and smoked cigars. He took naps in the late afternoon. He took calls and dictated letters while enjoying relaxing and prolonged baths.[20] Napping and bathing aside, I would advocate taking up some healthier habits. Still, the point is that even amidst the highest-order stress, what allows us to persevere is surrounding those challenging moments with habits that support our well-being. At least mental well-being, if not physical, in the case of Churchill.

So, take care of the basics and prioritize the fulfillment of your various hierarchy of needs. By doing so, you're stacking the deck in your favor each day, giving you an advantage over the stressors and anxieties that are eager to creep in. Reflect on what makes situations hard for you or where worry will most likely appear. Are there stressful experiences you just try to "get through" time and again, looking ahead to some future activity or reward? If so, maybe there's an opportunity to combine something you "have to do" with something you "want to do."

Consider the bad habits you want to replace and the triggers and cravings that perpetuate their continuation. Alternatively, what good habits have you always "wished" you could adopt? Could today be the day you give it a try? If so, be intentional about the key elements enabling your habit to stick, making it obvious, attractive, easy, and satisfying. Ensure those chosen habits are consistent with your identity, whether that identity is already engrained or if it's the one you choose for yourself moving forward. And focus on the process. What small things can you do each moment to the best of your abilities? Remember that presence and anxiety cannot coexist. Let the outcomes take care of themselves and direct your focus on what's in front of you. Before long, your hard work and discipline will have cultivated an environment that makes it easy to live with presence and rise above your past worries.

8.5 – The Bonus: How to Speak

This is your bonus chapter. Well, half-chapter. It's a half-chapter because its topic is more symptom than source, so I'm keeping it brief. Our focus has been on the core of your anxiety. Mastering your thoughts is the key to victory. But as we learned in Chapter 2, "*The Source of Anxiety & The Most Powerful Thought*," there's a difference between stress and anxiety. Even if lasting anxiety no longer plagues you, you'll still run into situations that trigger your stress response.

Also, while you can stand firmly against your *lasting* anxiety, there will be events that challenge your resolve and days when the pressures of life can still feel overwhelming. When you run into stress and anxiety, there will be physical symptoms of those feelings, like a more rapid heart rate, a tensing of your muscles and body, or a flushing of the skin or sweating. In Chapter 7, "*The Train Has Left the Station*," we talked about what to do when your anxious thoughts have already established momentum. Now, we'll dive deeper to address one issue of particular importance for most jobs today and many significant moments in our personal lives. That's the act of speaking.

Do you have situations where your heart races as you talk? Have you ever lost your breath while trying to get the words out? Has your mind "gone blank" as you suddenly forgot your planned words, and panic set in? The problem is likely to be the *way* that you're speaking. More precisely, the problem is how you *breathe* when speaking.

Some people call anxiety a breathing problem. That's not true; it's a thinking problem. But there's a reason why many make that claim, as irregular breathing patterns and a suboptimal breathing technique will have cascading effects. Remember that our heartbeat, blood circulation, and brain functioning rely on oxygen intake. When we don't breathe properly, we strain our system, impact our heart rate, and inhibit our ability to think clearly. Chapter 7 covered the importance of slow breathing through the nose. Most of the books on public speaking, and even those on the very topic of breathing, will detail breathing exercises to conduct *before* you speak. But what about our breathing *as* we speak?

Studies have shown that healthy adults are more likely to breathe through their noses at rest. That changes when we communicate. During speech, most people breathe through the nose *and* mouth.[1] When we're stressed or if we start to panic, we breathe irregularly, which can take different forms. Stress may cause us to unconsciously hold our breath, denying our body its required oxygen intake. However, the reverse can be true, as "panic breathing" typically involves rapid gulps of air through the mouth. This hyperventilation introduces too much oxygen that overwhelms our systems. In addition, air intake through the mouth is not filtered, it's not humidified, and its flow is harder to regulate. These drawbacks of mouth breathing are all benefits of breathing through the nose.

Why will our voice begin to fail us if we breathe through the mouth? It's because we're taking in this unfiltered, non-humidified air that dries out our vocal cords. Having recognized these facts about the benefits of nasal breathing when resting, I realized that when speaking, I most often relied on breath intake through my mouth. I started to notice the same pattern in most others and decided to experiment.

I switched from breathing through my mouth to exclusively breathing through my nose as I spoke. This change was a lot harder than you might think. I've probably been breathing when speaking the same way my entire life. It's an unconscious process. I had to make that process a conscious one for an extended period. It felt very awkward initially, both the process itself and the long pauses I perceived as I stopped speaking to breathe through my nose. As I practiced, I often felt the need to take a breath mid-sentence, which is the real cause of awkwardness in pauses. However, I very shortly saw the promise in the approach, and after several weeks, it transformed both my attitude and my performance in public speaking.

Here's how you can do the same. Practice by reading a book out loud. Do it with a strong voice. You're not whispering; you're projecting the words. You can try the technique with this very book, though be warned that, at first, you won't be absorbing the content of what you read, as your focus will be on the breathing method. If you have kids, reading aloud to them is a great option. The critical element, which will take some time to master, is *when* to take each breath and how big of a breath to take.

Taking a five-second breath in through the nose as you speak can yield an uncomfortably long pause, especially if taken at the wrong time. However, we don't need to fill our lungs to capacity with each breath. Use punctuation in the text to signal when you can breathe and how big of a breath that should be. A comma offers a chance to pause and take a small breath if you need one. A period is a signal to take a normal breath. A new paragraph allows you to take a full breath. If you follow these cues, those pauses will sound natural and benefit your speech (assuming what you're reading is structured well).

The breaks allow your audience the time to reflect on your message and process the information. The awkwardness only comes if you run out of breath and pause in the middle of a sentence. However, even in those circumstances, stay committed to breathing through your nose. Breathing through your nose will make it easier to recover if you start to get nervous, compared with when you're panic-breathing through your mouth. You're also likely to think you're pausing longer than you really are. Go ahead and record yourself as you're doing this reading practice. You'll notice that the pauses, which seem long and uncomfortable, aren't quite so apparent. And, when you successfully align your breaths with the punctuation, your speech will sound effective and purposeful.

Begin your practice by reading the book out loud, then extend the practice to conversations with your family and friends. After a few days, make the cutover at work. As you're speaking, breathe entirely through your nose without relying on air intake through your mouth.

Here's another secret to the morning ritual I didn't initially share when we discussed "*The Process*" in Chapter 3. As you're conducting your morning meeting or prayer to plan your daily thoughts, do it out loud. And I mean loud, with a strong speaking voice. Breathe in through your nose and speak out through your mouth your assessment of yesterday and your plan for the day ahead. If you can do it while conducting an aerobic activity such as walking or running, it will be powerful training for your speech, building your capacity to speak whole sentences from each breath through the nose. Your practice while at rest will feel easy by comparison.

Beyond conditioning your vocal strength, conducting your morning meeting aloud has a major added benefit. When you verbally declare your plan in the morning, the words will have greater resolve, resonance, and clarity. If you instead conduct your meeting entirely inside your head, your planning session risks being overtaken by a sea of competing thoughts. Communicate your daily plan audibly and with conviction. It will be far more likely to stick.

After a few weeks of practice, breathing through your nose during speech will become unconscious. You'll notice your voice becoming stronger. You won't have to clear your throat so often. Your vocal capacity will remain steady, even after prolonged periods of speaking. You won't run out of breath as your breathing will remain slow, controlled, and regulated through your speech. Most importantly, as you communicate, you'll feel a greater clarity of thought as your brain is delivered the oxygen it requires for proper function.

All these factors will result in speaking with greater poise and confidence. Fewer struggles and better performances will become a self-reinforcing system to propel you forward. So don't just commit to breathing *exercises* or focus on your breathing *before* the critical moments; transform your breathing *during* those moments. Breathe entirely through your nose. Speak as you exhale. Pause at the conclusion of your sentences to breathe again. As you do, you'll enjoy the benefits of that filtered, humidified air as it slowly enters your lungs, producing a strong voice, steady blood flow, and clear thinking.

Chapter Nine

Where Does Your Help Come From?

We have the power to control many of our thoughts, attitudes, and feelings, but can we self-help our way to *complete* freedom from anxiety? I believe the answer is "no." My opinion may come as a surprise, given we've focused on how to exert control over unconscious processes in the brain, the discipline needed to establish a system to shape our thoughts, and the importance of assuming extreme personal accountability. Yes, these are required practices to live every moment "wanting to be here," but we can't do it alone.

What won't be a surprise at this point in the book is that I have a strong faith in God. Whether you believe in God or not, consider the words of Psalm 23. Read these words slowly, "The Lord is my shepherd; I have all that I need. He lets me rest in green meadows; he leads me beside peaceful streams. He renews my strength. He guides me along right paths, bringing honor to his name. Even when I walk through the darkest valley, I will not be afraid, for you are close beside me. Your rod and your staff protect and comfort me. You prepare a feast for me in the presence of my enemies. You honor me by anointing my head with oil. My cup overflows with blessings. Surely your goodness and unfailing love will pursue me all the days of my life, and I will live in the house of the Lord forever."[1]

When stress overwhelms my process, when cracks in my inner strength challenge my discipline, and when anxieties overrun my control, I need a helper who allows me to "rest in green meadows." I need a presence to "renew my strength." I need to be led "beside peaceful streams." I won't turn this chapter into a sermon or push my faith on you. If you believe in God, lean into His strength. And whether you believe in God or not, where else can you turn for support? A therapist, a spouse, a close friend? My recommendation is simple: take extreme ownership of all the factors you have even a measure of control over in your life, and then also get help.

Sources of Help

In this book, we've focused on the factors you *can* control, but there are many influences we *can't* control that significantly impact our mental state and predispositions. Principal among those is our genetic makeup. No universally accepted ratio specifies the extent to which we are shaped by genetics and biology (nature) versus learned experience and environmental factors (nurture). The debate has been waged for centuries, dating back to Greek philosophers and likely long before. We can ramp up the "nurture" side of the equation through intention. However, even if we can tip the balance in favor of experience through focused effort, nature will always play a meaningful role in our personalities, behaviors, and tendencies.

While our genetics are unchanging, some aspects of "nurture" also remain fixed. None of the events and experiences from your childhood or past that have shaped your current inclinations, traits, and mental state will change. For me, there's a combination of my genetics and childhood experiences that predisposed me to panic attacks. Everyone has a past, and we've all faced trials that have shaped us, often unconsciously.

In the initial chapters, I was intentional in framing the "I don't want to be here" thought as the *source* of our anxiety but not as the *root cause*. To illustrate the difference, picture a garden. The gardener has the capacity to shape the outputs in the garden (the plants, the flowers, the vegetables) by watering the plants, pruning the leaves, and fertilizing the soil. We are the gardener. Our thoughts are the stems of the plants and flowers. Through our efforts, we can shape our thoughts to be healthy and constructive. Those positive thoughts will produce our desired feelings and actions, which are the plants' healthy fruits.

Yet, there's an unseen aspect to this picture. In the garden, there's still a reason those plants can grow in the first place that has nothing to do with soil, watering, or pruning. Those plants are there because, beneath the surface, there are roots, and those roots grew out of seeds. In the same way, the "I don't want to be here" thought has roots that grew from a seed. That seed is the root cause of your anxious feelings. It was planted through a combination of your genetics and any experiences or even traumas that shaped you.

Of course, nothing will alter what happened in your past, so you might as well accept it. But how can you accept a fact that sits just below your consciousness? Knowledge is power, and understanding how the past has shaped you can provide the insights you need to overcome the challenges you face. As Oprah Winfrey said in her book, *What Happened To You?*, "Your past is not an excuse, but it *is* an explanation, offering insight into the questions so many of us ask ourselves. Why do I behave the way I behave? Why do I feel the way I do?"[2] In the same way that the first step in eliminating a bad habit is to identify your habit's triggers, understanding the underlying forces that shape stress, anxiety, and other challenging feelings will help you to overcome them.

You've probably picked up that the "T" in CBT stands for "therapy." While the morning ritual of unpacking your behaviors from yesterday and identifying the thoughts that drove those actions can be a personal exercise, you will have blind spots that a neutral third party can help you uncover. We often hold negative thoughts deep inside, influencing our actions, which we don't want to admit to ourselves. Yet unless and until they're uncovered, we can't flip them. I've detailed some of those ugly thoughts I've had towards my own family. While I didn't want to admit they were there, I had to be honest about their presence to change them. My morning routine acts as a self-directed, daily CBT therapy session. The added benefit? Zero copays and no getting cut off because the next appointment has arrived.

Introspection should be a regular practice whether you see a therapist or not, but an outside perspective can help you do the hard work of identifying the root thoughts that you either can't see or can't bring yourself to see. The 2020 National Health Interview Survey, managed by the Centers for Disease Control or CDC, found that about 10% of adults in the U.S. received therapy or counseling treatment for their mental health in the past 12 months.[3] While the incidence of therapy is on the rise, most with an anxiety disorder forego this form of help. The National Institute for Mental Health estimates over 30% of U.S. adults experience an anxiety disorder at some point in their lives.[4] That's considering only disorders. How many people experience stress and anxiety that often feels overwhelming? *That* figure will be a lot closer to 100%. For some, there remains a stigma associated with therapy, particularly among men. We need to realize that seeking help is not a sign of weakness; it's a sign of intelligence.

Enlisting the help of a professional is a great option, as these impartial specialists are trained in the science that underpins our mental health. There are other options, though. Do you have someone you trust at work that you can confide in? What about a friend or family member? Talk with them about the thoughts fueling your anxieties. Chances are they'll have their own experience to draw from and a perspective to see things you cannot.

Oprah has been candid about the significant emotional and physical trauma she experienced as a child. She wrote the book mentioned earlier to describe how unpacking past events can help us better understand our current mental state. While she has never gone to official therapy, she describes daily conversations with one of her close friends as fulfilling that purpose.[2] I have the benefit of a great brother-in-law who is at once family, a close friend, and who happens to be a top-notch therapist specializing in CBT. While we've never done an official therapy session together, I can sense his tricks as we get deep into conversation. By bringing others into the problem-solving process, we gain knowledge and insights we would miss on our own.

Reading is another avenue to gain wisdom to combat stress and anxiety. I recommend every book I've cited in this text and much more. Before I made nonfiction reading and audiobooks an everyday habit, I asked my boss, who was going through a top MBA program at the time, which book I should read between the options of *The Innovator's Dilemma* and *Crossing the Chasm*, both seminal books in technology. I knew these books would take many hours to read; I believed I only had time for one, and I wanted to make the choice that would confer the greater benefit. He recommended *The Innovator's Dilemma*, but I didn't realize until after I had taken up my reading habit that the real answer was, "Read both... and read a whole lot more."

Now, with every book I read, I'm in search of even a single piece of wisdom I can apply to improve my performance at work, my approach at home, introduce a new technique, change my mindset, and more. I'll read in themes, covering a few books on a single or connected topic in succession to explore different angles. I spent hundreds of dollars every year on books (some of the best investments I have made), only to rediscover the library and that there is an endless supply of the books I had been paying for available in digital and audio copies for free. Building our knowledge base is how we gain strength, confidence, and prepare ourselves for life's challenges.

Substances to Help

From the CDC's 2020 National Health Interview Survey, I mentioned that about 10% of U.S. adults have leveraged therapy or counseling in the past year. That translates to tens of millions in the U.S. alone utilizing this form of assistance. However, what's far more prevalent is the incidence of adults relying on prescription medications to combat mental health challenges. The same survey found that the proportion of U.S. adults taking medication was 65% higher than that of those leveraging therapy and counseling. *Disclaimer: I am not a doctor. Make decisions about medications with a trained medical professional.* While I won't seek to influence any individual decision, there is a worrying trend when prescription medications (not even considering over-the-counter options) significantly outpace other forms of intervention.

Consider my personal example. I have a panic attack for the first time. I'm a physically fit person in my 20s. I undergo several tests which confirm my physical health. The doctor spends a few minutes with me, and I leave the hospital with a prescription for the anti-anxiety medication Prozac. I don't go to the doctor a lot, but I've also had knee injuries that led me to an orthopedic specialist. Visits to different doctors will all have their nuances. Still, although I could barely walk and my knee had swollen like a balloon, the doctor sent me home with a recommendation to do months of physical therapy before considering surgery. Her message was that invasive surgery could be avoided if I put in the work and implemented the proper techniques and exercises to strengthen the muscles supporting my knee.

Why are we often taking a different approach to our mental health than we would with our physical health? Drugs may be necessary, but they shouldn't be the first option. At my emergency room visit, not a single recommendation was made to change my diet, exercise regimen, or habits. I didn't come away with a book recommendation offering a new philosophy to change my mindset. I wasn't given a list of therapists I might consider. He didn't explain how the brain works and the processes that lead to anxiety and panic attacks. In his defense, I'm in an emergency room surrounded by others with (surprise) emergencies. I was physically "fine," and he needed to move on to the people with "real" issues. I may not have had a physical ailment, but my mind was not working the way that it should. I needed to build it up through strength and endurance training, as I would with my body. Not to mention the laundry list of possible side effects from these drugs. One of which for Prozac is anxiety![5]

Particularly for people who suffer from stress and anxiety, we need to be very careful about the substances we put in our bodies (hence the "extreme" diet that I practice). Take a more innocuous example of the caffeine in coffee. I've found an equal number of studies asserting the negative health impacts of coffee as those claiming that coffee will help you live to 100, so I'm not even going to go there in citing any research. Instead, let's focus on what caffeine does to our bodies. Yes, it releases feel-good hormones like dopamine, but it also releases adrenaline to amp us up, as well as cortisol, the stress hormone. When anxiety is creeping in, cortisol is already released unnecessarily into our bodies. There's a potential interaction effect that can have significant implications for those with anxiety. Independently, coffee can boost productivity, alertness, and mood. However, couple a little bit of the adrenaline and cortisol from coffee with a little bit of stress at work, and suddenly, the anxiety can turn overwhelming.

Coffee was a daily ritual for me. When I joined VMware, they had one of those fancy espresso machines, and I got into making iced espresso drinks. Sometimes, I'd have a couple during the day. What I noticed was that my anxiety was spiking in conjunction with the coffee consumption. If I experienced stress at work (which was pretty much every day) and I had coffee, then the anxiety symptoms, including worrying, heart racing, and tightness in my chest, would be accentuated.

The breakthrough in my understanding of the relationship actually came outside of work when I was shopping for diapers. If that sounds surprising, then you've never been in a store calculating how you're about to spend over a hundred dollars on a product that will soon be covered with human excrement. If that's not anxiety-inducing, I don't know what is. So, as I'm doing these calculations in my head, I feel the same symptoms of anxiety I've had at work. I look over accusingly at the iced coffee drink in my hand. The jig was up, and I knew it was to blame.

I cannot overstate the benefit that giving up caffeine has had on my ability to manage anxiety. The problem is that I drank coffee every day for years, and it was one of the small pleasures I looked forward to each morning. You might think you'll take a little added cortisol if the alternative is losing your favorite coffee habit. However, consider that through habit change and introducing replacements, you could have something you appreciate even more. A morning fruit smoothie has replaced my coffee habit and become even more enjoyable.

Now, before you stage a revolt because you think I'm coming after the best part of your morning, recognize that my message is to consider how different foods, drinks, or substances conspire to impact your mental state. Carefully observe any possible connections between what you consume and how you feel. If you don't perceive an association, keep doing what you're doing. However, if you think there could be a negative relationship between stress, anxiety, and caffeine (or something similar), experiment with different options. Maybe espresso is a no-go, but tea is fine. Or, if you find yourself inspired to jump into the life-changing world of cold showers, you will discover that cold water wakes you up much more effectively than any coffee. Perhaps a replacement "wakeup habit" frees you to try a decaffeinated option, allowing for the same tastes, smells, and experience without all the caffeine. The same relationships and experimentation should be observed and applied to other substances that impact your hormonal balance and may be interacting with stress to drive anxiety symptoms.

There are other non-prescription substances people will turn to with the express intention of reducing their anxiety. Highly prevalent are smoking and alcohol. Yet, these two have the same potential hormone production issue as we discussed with coffee. Yes, they release pleasure-inducing hormones that aid in relaxation. However, they are also both linked to the release of cortisol, which is the last thing you want to boost when your fight-or-flight response is already unhelpfully cranking the stress hormone out. The other implication, beyond the obvious downsides of smoking and drinking related to physical health, is we can build up a dependency. The mind is powerful, and we can start feeling like we "need" certain things to cope with stressful situations. When giving a presentation, for example, some people will "need" to have a glass of water or water bottle next to them, or they won't go through with it. It's a good idea to stay hydrated when you're speaking or need to clear your throat, but you don't want to build an unnecessary dependency.

I have a close friend I used to work with who had an interesting habit related to alcohol. We were discussing presentations and how to deal with nerves. He admitted that before every presentation, he would take a shot of peppermint schnapps alcohol. It both dealt with his nerves and freshened his breath simultaneously. We shared a good laugh at his tactic. But when I asked him if he really did it every time, he responded, "Yes, because it's worked before, so why risk not doing it?" My friend has gone on to a very successful career (and I confirmed he dropped the tactic), but at that time, he believed part of his success came from the alcohol. He was fully capable of succeeding without the "confidence boost," yet he had begun to develop a dependency.

With this example in mind, when I had the honor to deliver a "best man" wedding speech in front of hundreds of people, I intentionally avoided any sip of alcohol beforehand until the final moment of the toast, which concluded the speech. Why? I didn't want my crazy brain to think that I was only able to do it because I used a substance to calm my nerves in advance. I wanted the knowledge that I had done it with a clear mind and could do it again in any setting, work or social, without needing any substance.

Again, if you and your doctor agree on medication, that can be good. Different forms and intensity levels of anxiety require different interventions. Many forms are far more extreme than what I have experienced personally. In all cases, we should be discerning about the substances we put in our bodies to alter our mental states. When possible, exhaust the potential for natural remedies as a first option, particularly with children. The CDC study found that 6% of U.S. children aged 5 to 11 took prescription medication for mental health, with that figure increasing to 11% for those aged 12 to 17.[6] That is over 4 million U.S. kids going through significant developmental changes at the same time as taking mood-altering drugs. While therapy as a treatment option is more prevalent than medication for children, the gap between these approaches is slim for boys, who are significantly more likely than girls to be medicated and less likely to receive counseling.

Younger generations are struggling more. The Census Bureau's Household Pulse Survey in 2023 demonstrated a linear relationship between anxiety levels and generation, with half of those between the ages of 18 to 24 reporting symptoms of either an anxiety or depressive disorder, or both. In case you missed that, I said *one-half*. That compares to 38% for those 25 to 49 and 29% for those 50 to 64.[7] Research has shown that this tendency towards anxiety among the nation's youth is not just a matter of life-stage-related challenges, with Gen Z demonstrating higher levels of anxiety compared with Millennials at the same point in their lives.[8]

Humans have gone through hundreds of thousands of years without relying on these mind-altering medications to the degree we do today. Although there is evidence of medicinal plant use that predates the onset of farming as humans practiced hunter-gathering lifestyles, the first antipsychotic and antidepressant medications weren't introduced until the 1950s.[9] Alongside the rise in mental health medications has come an increase in the prevalence of anxiety itself. Shouldn't we see a *decrease* in mental health issues if the intervention of these drugs is so helpful?

As a society, we are relying on drugs and abdicating our responsibilities for education. When you are a hammer, every problem looks like a nail. For the pharmaceutical industry, every mental health issue is a nail to be solved by the hammer of their prescriptions. The problem is growing, and we need (and our youth needs) education on how to take control of our mental health. We can all build mental strength and resilience through intention, dedication, and the application of knowledge in how anxiety forms and what to do to combat it.

***

We're living in a world where the prevalence of anxiety is growing. There are many additional factors that we haven't explored that conspire to fuel anxious thinking. Some of the big ones include the overuse of social media, constant attention on negativity in the news cycle, and the long-term shift in society towards isolation. These external factors and stimuli are coupled with personal dynamics like our genetics, our past experiences, and any trauma we may have faced, particularly in childhood.

The system described in this book is a powerful method for taking control of your mental health. You can and should take ownership of every factor that contributes to your anxiety that is within your control. But also be humble enough to realize that you need help, because we all do. Be cautious and thoughtful when it comes to the substances intended to help us relax or otherwise alter our mental state, ranging from relatively innocuous options like caffeine to prescription medications. Establish support sources beyond substances, including faith, family, friends, community, and therapy.

Chapter Ten

Conclusion

I started with a story, and I'll end with a story. But while the opening story was about me, the closing one is about you. You picked up this book because some form of stress and anxiety has been overstepping its bounds, standing in the way of the life you want to live. The anxieties have built up until they've burst, with physical implications and mental spiraling. You've been waking up each morning with a weight on your shoulders. You've said 'no' to opportunities at work for fear of not living up to your potential. You've had too many 'mostly good days' with your significant other or kids, where you lost your patience just momentarily, and a few moments of stress-fueled anger and frustration ruined hours of positive interactions. You've spent time worrying that you're not qualified for the job you have, fearing your lack of knowledge will be "exposed." You've too often let the anxieties of what you "have to do" next cause you to miss the special moments happening right now. You've sat through too many meetings without participating, counting the minutes until it was over, yet with simultaneous apprehension that you'll be unwillingly brought into the conversation. You've endlessly ruminated on what others have done wrong and have even had full arguments with them staged entirely in your mind. You've taken on too many tasks against your will, overloading yourself and resenting the burden you "have to" carry. You've accepted your negative habits and put off the beneficial ones you've longed to adopt. You spend too much of each day not wanting to be where you are.

But today is a new day. You wake up and decide that the most important meeting you'll have is the one with yourself. As you prepare for what's ahead, you identify in advance the situations that tripped you up the day before. You retrain the thoughts in you that color your negative interactions, repeating and readying your replacement thoughts for when they are needed. You commit that in each interaction to come, you will show up with an attitude of "I want to be here." You decide to be intentional about how you spend your time today. For every planned activity, you reflect on the *thinking purpose* and the *feeling purpose* driving each, ensuring you have logical and emotional drivers underpinning how you spend your time. When you identify a flimsy purpose or none at all, you resolve to remove or replace that activity. You decide today will be the day you introduce a new habit you've wanted to implement for years. You start slowly and in increments, trusting that momentum will build if you take the first small step.

At work, you eliminate the non-essentials. You decline a meeting where you're unlikely to make an impact. You avoid the distraction of lower-priority e-mails and instant messages, focusing instead on the 20% of activities that will generate 80% of your results. Where you choose to participate – the meetings, the discussions, the hallway conversations – you lean in 100%. You want to be there. You engage. You recognize you are there for a reason and commit to making your presence felt. No one can put you on the spot because you've proactively stepped onto the center stage. You re-energize yourself through the day with healthy food, exercise, and activities you enjoy. You prioritize the time with your family, being fully present in the moments you share. You look them in the eyes to keep your mind from wandering. You see them and appreciate what's happening at each moment.

As you inevitably face hurdles during the day and stress and anxiety begin to creep in, you call a timeout. You focus on your breathing. You observe the negative thoughts forming in you and recognize the forces in your brain that have cultivated their arrival. You rely on the support of a trusted friend or family member. Then, you get off the sideline and back in the game. You repeat the replacement thoughts you practiced in advance and know to be true. And when your thoughts aren't enough, you flip the paradigm and leverage your actions to inspire the right thoughts. Even when you don't feel like it, you choose to engage in a positive activity and leave your brain no choice but to come along for the ride, bringing the right feelings and thoughts with it. You answer the higher call, stepping into a situation with your family or your teammates charged with stress. You deploy the power of your thoughts to deliver calm during the storm and allow your peace to permeate the room. You realize that the thoughts you've been repeating all day are not a mental trick but your reality. You are genuinely thankful for each interaction, each opportunity, and each engagement. You chose to be there. The thought now comes to you spontaneously, and you know it to be true. You hear the words ringing in your mind: "I want to be here."

Acknowledgments

With books and audiobooks, I often continue reading or listening through the acknowledgments section out of curiosity. It's interesting to hear the people thanked, but I often wondered how much an author's family or friends contributed to the final product. I learned a key lesson through writing this book. It's not that you divvy up the chapters and everyone writes one; it's the value of the different perspectives. And in what was an especially happy surprise, everyone brought something unique. Those insights made the book immeasurably better than it would or could have been if written from only my perspective. Writing this book and receiving feedback deepened my appreciation for the importance of diversity of thought in creating something [hopefully] of value.

My father-in-law, Jim Winston, showed me the importance of telling a good story. The great therapist, friend, and brother-in-law I mentioned, Ben Leahy, helped shape many of the psychological concepts and draw out new insights. The feedback from my friend and former coworker, Chris Norton, made the book more inclusive, and he provided loads of practical advice through multiple rounds of revision. My sister, Jamie Leahy, offered the eye of the skilled educator that she is to supply a layer of polish. My teammate, Yucy Fang, helped make the premise more expansive and brought an essential point of view of how women in the workplace experience anxiety. As a bonus, she also designed an incredible book cover. My Mom, Holly Seaver, helped connect the loose ends to ensure I finished strong. And the conversations with my friends, Jeff O'Connor, Matt Plicque, Stephen Chan, and Steve Tettke, provided vital redirection and support throughout the project. Thank you to each of you for reading versions of the book that I would now be embarrassed to share and helping to shape it into something much better.

To my family: my son, Colby, thank you for sitting next to me night after night as we both did our "work," with me writing and you playing your math game on your laptop. Colby, as well as my son Caleb and daughter Eliana, thank you for inspiring many of the stories in the book, but more importantly, for inspiring my desire to be present, to show up as my best for you, and to appreciate all that you do in each stage of life (even the splashes of bathwater to the face). And to my wife, Suzy, my partner in all things: thank you for your continual support, for not letting that stop you from telling it to me straight, and for being my motivation to think the right thoughts.

Notes

Chapter 1

1. Psychology Today. (2019). *Imposter syndrome*. Psychology Today. https://www.psychologytoday.com/us/basics/imposter-syndrome

2. Dwyer, Karen & Davidson, Marlina. (2012). *Is Public Speaking Really More Feared Than Death?*. Communication Research Reports. 29. 99-107. 10.1080/08824096.2012.667772.

Chapter 2

1. Villines, Z. (2022, May 19). *Eustress vs. distress: Difference, examples, and effects*. Www.medicalnewstoday.com. https://www.medicalnewstoday.com/articles/eustress-vs-distress#comparison

2. Barrell, A. (2020). *Stress vs. anxiety: Differences, symptoms, and relief*. Www.medicalnewstoday.com. https://www.medicalnewstoday.com/articles/stress-vs-anxiety

3. National Institute of Mental Health. (2023). *The Teen brain: 7 Things to Know.* National Institute of Mental Health. https://www.nimh.nih.gov/health/publications/the-teen-brain-7-things-to-know

4. Cleveland Clinic. (2022, March 30). *Brain: Anatomy, Development and Function.* Cleveland Clinic; Cleveland Clinic. https://my.clevelandclinic.org/health/body/22638-brain

5. Cleveland Clinic. (2022, May 23). *Cerebral Cortex.* Cleveland Clinic. https://my.clevelandclinic.org/health/articles/23073-cerebral-cortex

6. Shapiro, J. (2021, November 5). *Two Parts of the Brain Govern Much of Mental Life | Psychology Today.* Www.psychologytoday.com. https://www.psychologytoday.com/us/blog/thinking-in-black-white-and-gray/202111/two-parts-the-brain-govern-much-mental-life

7. Drucker, P. F. (1959). *Landmarks of Tomorrow: a report on the new "post-modern" world.* Transaction Publishers.

8. Murphy, T. F. (2021, October 3). *Cognitive Behavioral Therapy.* Psychology Fanatic. https://psychologyfanatic.com/cognitive-behavioral-therapy/

9. *Tom Brady's Mental Toughness: The 4 Principles He Relies On.* (n.d.). TB12. https://tb12sports.com/blogs/tb12/tom-bradys-mental-toughness

10. *English Standard Version Bible.* (2016). Crossway Bibles.

11. Allen, J. (2019). *As A Man Thinketh.* Indoeuropeanpublishing Co.

12. *Top 10 Marcus Aurelius Quotes.* (2023, December 7). Stoic Simple |. https://www.stoicsimple.com/top-10-marcus-aurelius-stoic-quotes-famous-stoicism-meditations/

13. (2006, June 23). *Click* (J. Gourson, Ed.) [DVD Click]. Columbia Pictures.

14. Dr. Marques, L. (2023). *Bold Move.* HarperOne.

Chapter 3

1. Burgess, L. (2018, February 27). *What percentage of our brain do we use?* Medicalnewstoday.com; Medical News Today. https://www.medicalnewstoday.com/articles/321060#how-much-of-our-brain-do-we-use

2. Young, E. (2018, July 25). *Lifting the lid on the unconscious.* New Scientist. https://www.newscientist.com/article/mg23931880-400-lifting-the-lid-on-the-unconscious/

3. Goggins, D. (2022). *Never Finished.* Lioncrest Publishing.

4. *A-Rod admits taking PEDs during 3-year period.* (2009, February 9). ESPN.com. https://www.espn.com/mlb/news/story?id=3894847

5. Tworek, G. (2023, December 12). *What Is Neuroplasticity? How It Works.* Cleveland Clinic. https://health.cleveland clinic.org/neuroplasticity

6. Dweck, C. (2012). *Mindset: How You Can Fulfil Your Potential.* Constable & Robinson.

Chapter 4

1. WFAA. (2024, June 25). *1992 United States presidential debate | Bill Clinton, George H.W. Bush, Ross Perot.* YouTube. https://www.youtube.com/watch?v=DidJk3D1RaI

2. *Bush vs. Dukakis: The second 1988 presidential debate.* (n.d.). Www.youtube.com. https://www.youtube.com/watch?v=hHCUvx3tpnM

3. *President George H.W. Bush Interview | Debating Our Destiny* | April 10, 1999 | PBS. (2024). Pbs.org . https://www.pbs.org/newshour/spc/debatingourdestiny/interviews/bush.html

4. Madore KP, Wagner AD. *Multicosts of Multitasking.* Cerebrum. 2019 Apr 1;2019:cer-04-19. PMID: 32206165; PMCID: PMC7075496.

5. Insurance Institute for Highway Safety. (2019). *Distracted driving.* IIHS-HLDI Crash Testing and Highway Safety. https://www.iihs.org/topics/distracted-driving

6. *76% of Employees Get More Distracted on Video Calls vs. In-person Meetings.* (n.d.). Showpad. https://www.showpad.com/press/76-of-employees-get-more-distracted-on-video-calls-vs-in-person-meetings/

7. *Virtual And Zoom Meeting Distraction Statistics [Survey] – Zippia.* (n.d.). https://www.zippia.com/advice/virtual-meetings-zoom-survey/

8. Bailenson, J. N. (2021). *Nonverbal Overload: A Theoretical Argument for the Causes of Zoom Fatigue.* Technology, Mind, and Behavior, 2(1). https://doi.org/10.1037/tmb0000030

Chapter 5

1. Isaacson, W. (2023). *Elon Musk.* Simon & Schuster.

2. Greg McKeown. (2014). *Essentialism : the disciplined pursuit of less.* Virgin Books.

3. Ferriss, T. (2007). *The 4-hour work week.* Vermilion.

4. Mandela, N. (1994). *Long Walk to Freedom : the Autobiography of Nelson Mandela.* Paw Prints. (Original work published 1994)

5. The Myers-Briggs Company. (2020, January 1). *How many introverted types are in leadership? World Introvert Day 2020.*

YouTube. https://www.youtube.com/watch?v=re4_Q2BgWxQ

6. Kennedy, J. F. (1962, September 12). *John F. Kennedy Address at Rice University*. Rice University. https://www.rice.edu/kennedy

7. Byerly, J. (2017, November 4). *The Janitor Who Helped Put a Man on the Moon*. From the Green Notebook. https://fromthegreennotebook.com/2017/11/04/the-janitor-who-help-put-a-man-on-the-moon/

8. X, M., & Haley, A. (2015). *The Autobiography of Malcolm X*. Ballantine Books. (Original work published 1965)

Chapter 6

1. Hatfield, E., Bensman, L., Thornton, P. D., & Rapson, R. L. (2014). *New Perspectives on Emotional Contagion: A Review of Classic and Recent Research on Facial Mimicry and Contagion*. Interpersona: An International Journal on Personal Relationships, 8(2), 159-179. https://doi.org/10.5964/ijpr.v8i2.162

2. *Final Programmatic Damage Assessment and Restoration Plan and Final Programmatic Environmental Impact Statement page 2-1 2. Incident Overview*. (n.d.) . https://www.gulfspillrestoration.noaa.gov/media/document/chapter-2incident-overview508pdf

3. Pallardy, R. (2024). *Deepwater Horizon oil spill.* In Encyclopaedia Britannica. https://www.britannica.com/event/Deepwater-Horizon-oil-spill

4. Walsh, B. (2010, July 25). Oil Spill: Goodbye, Mr. Hayward. Time. https://science.time.com/2010/07/25/oil-spill-goodbye-mr-hayward/

5. Korosec, K. (2010, April 29). Gulf Oil Spill: BP CEO Hayward Just Can't Help Blaming Someone Else. Www.cbsnews.com. https://www.cbsnews.com/news/gulf-oil-spill-bp-ceo-hayward-just-cant-help-blaming-someone-else/

6. *Chairman Waxman Questions BP CEO Tony Hayward.* (n.d.). Www.youtube.com. https://www.youtube.com/watch?v=Yj3ULzWpqt0

7. ABC News. (2010, July 26). *Tony Hayward's Failed Leadership*. YouTube. https://www.youtube.com/watch?v=jPfl61hwaEw

8. Lee, J. (2010, June 16). *President Obama's Oval Office Address on the BP Oil Spill: "A Faith in the Future that Sustains us as a People."* Whitehouse.gov. https://obamawhitehouse.archives.gov/blog/2010/06/16/president-obamas-oval-office-address-bp-oil-spill-a-faith-future-sustains-us-a-peopl

9. Mccarten, A. (2017). *Darkest hour : how Churchill brought us back from the brink*. Viking.

10. Churchill, W. (1940, June 4). *We Shall Fight on the Beaches - The International Churchill Society*. The International Churchill Society; Churchill. https://winstonchurchill.org/resources/speeches/1940-the-finest-hour/we-shall-fight-on-the-beaches/

11. *Winston Churchill "Blood, Toil, Tears and Sweat."* (2013). [YouTube Video]. In YouTube. https://www.youtube.com/watch?v=8TlkN-dcDCk

12. Greene, R. (1998). *The 48 Laws of Power*. Profile.

13. Kennedy, B. (2022). *Good Inside*. HarperCollins.

14. Willink, J., & Babin, L. (2015). *Extreme Ownership: How U.S. Navy SEALs Lead and Win*. Macmillan.

Chapter 7

1. American Psychiatric Association . (2020, March 5). *Psychiatry.org - Rumination: A Cycle of Negative Thinking*. Www.psychiatry.org . https://www.psychiatry.org/News-room/APA-Blogs/Rumination-A-Cycle-of-Negative-Thinking

2. Roland-Garros. (2020, June 6). *Graf vs Hingis 1999 Women's final Full Match | Roland-Garros*. YouTube. https://www.youtube.com/watch?v=py0BAzQC-Ts

3. *Martina Hingis | Biography, Titles, & Facts*. (n.d.). Ency-

clopedia Britannica. https://www.britannica.com/biography/Martina-Hingis

4. Staff Reporter. (2000, May 25). *"I think I lost my mind."* The Mail & Guardian. https://mg.co.za/article/2000-05-26-i-think-i-lost-my-mind/

5. Taylor, J., & Demick, A. (1994). *A multidimensional model of momentum in sports.* Journal of Applied Sport Psychology, 6(1), 51–70. https://doi.org/10.1080/10413209408406465

6. *An Examination of Timeout Value, Strategy, and Momentum in NCAA Division 1 Men's Basketball | USPROC.* (2019). Causeweb.org. https://www.causeweb.org/usproc/eusrc/2019/program/2

7. Permutt, S. (2011). *The Efficacy of Momentum-Stopping Timeouts on Short-Term Performance in the National Basketball Association.* TriCollege Libraries Institutional Scholarship. https://scholarship.tricolib.brynmawr.edu/server/api/core/bitstreams/c13af59d-819a-457e-8be5-6fb978264a2f/content

8. *In the dark for 34 minutes: The inside story of when the lights went out at the Super Bowl.* (2022, November 7). ESPN.com. https://www.espn.com/nfl/story/_/id/34946687/inside-ravens-49ers-2013-new-orleans-super-bowl-blackout

9. Nestor, J. (2020). *Breath: The new science of a lost art.* River-

head Books.

10. Johansen, L. (2010). *George Foreman vs Muhammad Ali - Oct. 30, 1974 - Entire fight - Rounds 1 - 8 & Interview*. In YouTube. https://www.youtube.com/watch?v=55AasOJZzDE

11. *George Foreman on why Muhammad Ali was so much more than a "boxer."* (2016, June 4). Shortlist. https://www.shortlist.com/news/george-foreman-on-ali

12. *In His Own Words - Muhammad Ali Center*. (2023, September 1). Alicenter.org. https://alicenter.org/meet-ali/in-his-own-words/

Chapter 8

1. Tyndale House Foundation. (2015). *Holy Bible: New Living Translation*. Tyndale House Publishers. (Original work published 1996)

2. *Is Being "Hangry" Really a Thing — or Just an Excuse?* (2021, June 7). Cleveland Clinic. https://health.clevelandclinic.org/is-being-hangry-really-a-thing-or-just-an-excuse

3. Danziger, S., Levav, J., & Avnaim-Pesso, L. (2011). *Extraneous factors in judicial decisions*. Proceedings of the National Academy of Sciences, 108(17), 6889–6892. https://doi.org/10.1073/pnas.1018033108

4. *The brain puts the memories warehouse in order while we sleep.* (n.d.). ScienceDaily. https://www.sciencedaily.com/releases/2018/03/180315110640.htm

5. Charest, J., & Grandner, M. A. (2020). *Sleep and Athletic Performance: Impacts on Physical Performance, Mental Performance, Injury Risk and Recovery, and Mental Health.* Sleep medicine clinics, 15(1), 41–57. https://doi.org/10.1016/j.jsmc.2019.11.005

6. Okano, K., Kaczmarzyk, J.R., Dave, N. et al. *Sleep quality, duration, and consistency are associated with better academic performance in college students.* npj Sci. Learn. 4, 16 (2019). https://doi.org/10.1038/s41539-019-0055-z

7. Thompson, J. (2022, March 14). *Tom Brady: 8 rules he followed to dominate the NFL.* Business Insider; Insider. https://www.businessinsider.com/diet-and-lifestyle-rules-tom-brady-followed-tol-2022-2#brady-goes-to-bed-at-830-pm-every-night-to-ensure-9-hours-of-sleep-1

8. News, A. B. C. (2023, December 30). *LeBron James turns 39: Here are 3 evidence-based approaches he uses to stay fit.* ABC News. https://abcnews.go.com/Sports/lebron-james-turns-39-evidence-based-approaches-he-uses-stay-fit/story?id=105844892

9. (2025). Somneesleep.com. *Sleep Habits 7 Olympic Athletes Use to Power Their Wins.* https://somneesleep.com/blogs

/post/7-olympic-athlete-sleep-habits-tips

10. Gorvett, Z. (n.d.). *What you can learn from Einstein's quirky habits.* Www.bbc.com . https://www.bbc.com/future/article/20170612-what-you-can-learn-from-einsteins-quirky-habits

11. Cleveland Clinic. (2022, February 23). *Hormones: What They Are, Function & Types.* Cleveland Clinic. https://my.clevelandclinic.org/health/articles/22464-hormones

12. Huberman, A. (2022, May 1). *The Science & Use of Cold Exposure for Health & Performance - Huberman Lab.* Www.hubermanlab.com. https://www.hubermanlab.com/newsletter/the-science-and-use-of-cold-exposure-for-health-and-performance

13. Tillage, R. P., Wilson, G. E., Liles, L. C., Holmes, P. V., & Weinshenker, D. (2020). *Chronic Environmental or Genetic Elevation of Galanin in Noradrenergic Neurons Confers Stress Resilience in Mice.* The Journal of neuroscience : the official journal of the Society for Neuroscience, 40(39), 7464–7474. https://doi.org/10.1523/JNEUROSCI.0973-20.2020

14. Cleveland Clinic. (2023, August 18). *What Is Your Gut Microbiome?* Cleveland Clinic. https://my.clevelandclinic.org/health/body/25201-gut-microbiome

15. *Conversation: Gut Feeling.* (2023, July 3). Uclahealth.org;

UCLA Health. https://www.uclahealth.org/news/publication/conversation-gut-feeling

16. *New study shows that diet has major impact on gut biomes.* (2021, March 23). Harvard Gazette. https://news.harvard.edu/gazette/story/2021/03/new-study-shows-that-diet-has-major-impact-on-gut-biomes/

17. Clear, J. (2018). *Atomic Habits: An Easy & Proven Way to Build Good Habits & Break Bad Ones.* Penguin Publishing Group.

18. Talty, J. (2022). *The leadership secrets of Nick Saban / How Alabama's coach became the greatest ever.* Matt Holt Books, An Imprint Of Benbella Books, Inc.

19. Patricia Ryan Madson. (2005). *Improv wisdom: don't prepare, just show up.* Bell Tower, Cop.

20. Mccarten, A. (2017). *Darkest hour : how Churchill brought us back from the brink.* Viking.

Chapter 8.5

1. Lester, R. A., & Hoit, J. D. (2014). *Nasal and oral inspiration during natural speech breathing.* Journal of speech, language, and hearing research : JSLHR, 57(3), 734–742. https://doi.org/10.1044/1092-4388(2013/13-0096)

Chapter 9

1. Tyndale House Foundation. (2015). *Holy Bible: New Living Translation.* Tyndale House Publishers. (Original work published 1996)

2. Oprah Winfrey, & Perry, B. (2021). *WHAT HAPPENED TO YOU? : conversations on trauma, resilience and healing.* Bluebird.

3. Terlizzi, E. P., & Norris, T. (2021, December 7). *Mental Health Treatment Among Adults: United States, 2020.* Products - Data Briefs - Number 419 - October 2021. Www.cdc.gov. https://www.cdc.gov/nchs/products/databriefs/db419.htm

4. National Institute of Mental Health. (2024). *Any Anxiety Disorder.* Www.nimh.nih.gov; National Institute of Mental Health. https://www.nimh.nih.gov/health/statistics/any-anxiety-disorder

5. WebMD. (2019). *Drugs & Medications.* Webmd.com . https://www.webmd.com/drugs/2/drug-6997/prozac-oral/details

6. Zablotsky, B., & Terlizzi, E. (2020, September 29). *Mental health treatment among children aged 5–17 years: United states, 2019.* Www.cdc.gov. https://www.cdc.gov/nchs/products/databriefs/db381.htm

7. Chris Lee. (2023, March 20). *Latest Federal Data Show*

That Young People Are More Likely Than Older Adults to Be Experiencing Symptoms of Anxiety or Depression. KFF. https://www.kff.org/mental-health/press-release/latest-federal-data-show-that-young-people-are-more-likely-than-older-adults-to-be-experiencing-symptoms-of-anxiety-or-depression/

8. Annie E. Casey Foundation. (2021, March 3). *Generation Z's Mental Health Issues - The Annie E. Casey Foundation*. The Annie E. Casey Foundation. https://www.aecf.org/blog/generation-z-and-mental-health

9. Hardy K. (2021). *Paleomedicine and the Evolutionary Context of Medicinal Plant Use*. Revista brasileira de farmacognosia : orgao oficial da Sociedade Brasileira de Farmacognosia, 31(1), 1–15. https://doi.org/10.1007/s43450-020-00107-4

Author Information

- E-mail: colemaninsightsink@gmail.com
- Facebook: www.facebook.com/colemaninsightsink
- LinkedIn: www.linkedin.com/in/1joecoleman

Made in USA - Kendallville, IN
39156_9798991918510
08.19.2025 2046